Not of Woman Born

Not of Woman Born

*Representations of Caesarean Birth
in Medieval and Renaissance Culture*

Renate Blumenfeld-Kosinski

Cornell University Press

ITHACA AND LONDON

First published 1990 by Cornell University Press.

International Standard Book Number 0-8014-2292-2
Library of Congress Catalog Card Number 89-17421

Printed in the United States of America.

Librarians: Library of Congress cataloging information appears on the last page of the book.

⊗ The paper used in this publication meets the minimum requirements of the American National Standard for Permanence of Paper for Printed Library Materials Z39.48-1984.

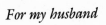
For my husband

CONTENTS

ACKNOWLEDGMENTS

This book took shape over many years, and along the way many people and institutions helped see it to its completion. I am grateful to Danielle Jacquart for encouraging me to turn an iconographic study of Caesarean birth into a cultural history of the operation. My special thanks go to George Saliba, who translated Arabic medical treatises for me far beyond the call of duty; the discussions we had on their interpretation made me see things in a new light. Luke Demaitre generously supplied as yet unpublished material on Bernard of Gordon's *Practica sive lilium medicinae*—on extremely short notice and at a crucial point in my research. Adelaide Bennett kindly shared her vast knowledge of medieval manuscript illuminations with me. Antoni Kosinski contributed some bibliographical detective work on medieval block books, the results of which are evident in Chapter 4. Kevin Brownlee and David Damrosch not only discussed the ramifications of my topic over several years, they also read the manuscript in an earlier version and made valuable suggestions that helped me reshape the entire work. The readers for Cornell University Press, as well, were generous with detailed suggestions. I thank all of them for the hard work they put into my manuscript. My thanks also go to Jean-Claude Schmitt, Dwayne Carpenter, and Margaret Schleissner, who were always alert for material relating to my study; to Richard Palmer from the Wellcome Library for tracking down elusive information; to Peter Jones from King's College Library in Cambridge for identifying an uncaptioned illustration from a medical "picture book"; and to the staff of the Interlibrary Loan Office at Columbia University, whose persistence and ingenuity made some strange and rare books available to me.

Several summer grants from the Columbia University Council for Research in the Humanities as well as a summer stipend from the National Endowment for the Humanities enabled me to do the necessary research in European libraries. I thank the staff of the Bibliothèque Nationale and the Bibliothèque de l'Arsenal in Paris, the Musée Condé in Chantilly, the British Library and the Wellcome Library for the History of Medicine in London, the Princeton University Library, the New York Public Library, the Pierpont Morgan Library in New York, and the Württembergische Landesbibliothek in Stuttgart, as well as the many libraries and collectors who supplied photographs and granted me permission to reproduce them.

Part of Chapter 4 has appeared in a slightly different version as "Illustration as Commentary in Late Medieval Images of Antichrist's Birth," in *Deutsche Vierteljahrsschrift für Literaturwissenschaft und Geistesgeschichte* 63:4 (1989).

Bernhard Kendler from Cornell University Press believed in this book from the beginning and saw it through the many steps from first draft to published book—my deep thanks go to him. To my husband, Antoni Kosinski, I dedicate this book. Without him and the countless ways in which he showed his support and enthusiasm it would never have seen the light of day.

RENATE BLUMENFELD-KOSINSKI

New York, N.Y.

Not of Woman Born

INTRODUCTION

"Not of woman born," "the Fortunate," "the Unborn"—the terms designating those born by Caesarean section in medieval and Renaissance Europe were mysterious and ambiguous. In antiquity, children fortunate enough to have survived a Caesarean birth were believed to be marked for a special destiny. Virgil describes one of them in the *Aeneid*: "Aeneas next kills Lichas, who had been cut out of his dead mother's womb and then made sacred, Phoebus unto you, because you let his infant life escape the knife."[1] Because he lived through his earliest encounter with the knife, Lichas was consecrated to Apollo; but he was fated to lose his life by this same instrument. By linking the moments of Lichas's birth and death, Virgil dramatizes the profound ambiguity surrounding both Caesarean birth itself and those born by it: their birth involves both mutilation and salvation. This twofold vision also informs medieval and Renaissance thought on Caesarean birth. At a time when a Caesarean was performed only if the mother died during labor, the child could indeed be considered as "not of woman born," or even "unborn," as signaled by the name "Nonnatus" or "Ingenito," given to a child born by Caesarean in tenth-century Germany.[2] Cut out of the womb, or "untimely ripp'd" as Shakespeare put it in *Macbeth* (act 5, scene 8), the newborn was the child not of a living woman but of a corpse.[3]

Was an unnatural coming into the world to be interpreted as a stigma or a good omen? According to Pliny's *Natural History* (7.9), birth by Caesarean was an auspicious omen for the child's future. This opinion was shared by a father in 1601 who gave the surname "Fortunatus" to his son born by Caesarean.[4] But for the mothers of these "fortunate" children Caesarean birth meant death and not life.

Over the centuries, attitudes toward Caesarean birth have been ambiguous because of its dual nature: meant to be life-giving, it was also life-threatening. With their mothers dead, not many newborns survived a delivery by Caesarean section for more than the moment it took to baptize them. Caesarean section was always an act of desperation.

Given the dramatic circumstances of most Caesarean births, it is not surprising that the operation was invested with many mythical beliefs and superstitions. Like some diseases the Middle Ages considered mysterious and incurable (leprosy comes to mind here),[5] Caesarean birth transcends the purely medical sphere and therefore becomes an ideal focal point for an exploration of important areas of medieval and Renaissance mentality. To reflect its multifaceted nature, not only must Caesarean birth be analyzed from a medical perspective, but it must also be linked to a theological and symbolic dimension.

No other medical procedure was so directly linked to spiritual salvation or damnation: as we will see, midwives were required by the church authorities to perform Caesareans if they believed a fetus may have been still alive after the mother's death; the goal was baptism and thus the salvation of the child. At the same time, Caesarean birth formed part of the controversy over which medical procedures midwives were allowed to perform. Thus the two crucial issues that distinguished Caesarean birth from normal childbirth, and that brought to a head questions of competency not at issue in regular obstetrics, were the frequent necessity for midwives to perform emergency baptism and the midwives' use of surgical instruments.

The Caesarean operation was seen as partaking simultaneously of the natural, the unnatural, and even the supernatural. This view of Caesarean birth determined many of its symbolic aspects; thus, in the Middle Ages, saints as well as devils were believed to have performed Caesareans.

Questions relating to the operation seldom have clear-cut answers. In the past, as today, Caesarean birth was caught in a tangle of ideological, political, and legal issues.[6] Who, for example, would decide that the mother was dead so that a Caesarean could be performed? Who was allowed to perform the operation? What were the consequences of hesitating too long or of a precipitous decision? How could the mother's or the child's spiritual salvation be assured? Were there any texts that could provide answers to such questions? And what can we know altogether about the performance of Caesarean sections in an age for which evidence even about normal childbirth is very scarce?

These are some of the questions I seek to answer in this book. In order to give the most comprehensive picture possible of Caesarean birth, I have centered the chapters of this book on the major types of sources that describe and depict the operation: medical, religious, and historical texts and documents as well as manuscript illuminations (for Caesar's birth) and woodcuts (for the Antichrist's birth by Caesarean). Thus the evidence concerning Caesarean birth comes from many disparate areas. Literature and mythology can give us some insight into medieval and Renaissance ideas and representations of Caesarean birth.[7] Medical and legal texts offer additional information. But the most fruitful source proves to be the iconography of Caesarean birth. Largely unexplored up to now, the iconographic tradition allows a study of the operation over several centuries and reveals some dramatic changes in its performance.

Most of the illuminations come from the *Faits des Romains* and French translations of Caesar's *Commentaries*.[8] Can such learned and literary sources provide evidence about "real" Caesarean sections?[9] I believe they can, for the study of the tradition of Caesarean birth in medical texts (Chapter 1) reveals a striking chronological coincidence between developments in these texts and those in the iconography (studied in Chapter 2): the first image appeared about 1300 in a Parisian manuscript; the first mention of Caesarean section in Western medicine appeared in 1305 in the *Practica sive lilium medicinae* by Bernard of Gordon, a physician from Montpellier. And about the time when female midwives were replaced by male surgeons in scenes of Caesarean birth, male medical writers began to describe their own experiences in performing the operation that previously only midwives had performed. Thus one of the most important conclusions of my study, the early marginalization of midwives in Caesarean births, can be documented in several areas simultaneously. But it is not enough to declare that marginalization took place; we also have to inquire into its possible origins. This is the focal point of Chapter 3.

Chapters 1 through 3 illuminate Caesarean birth from a variety of perspectives. In each chapter the operation is placed in a historical context. Thus, one of the focal points of Chapter 1 is the emergence of Caesarean birth in medical writings about 1305. A short analysis of attitudes toward pregnancy and birth opens the chapter. Since Caesarean section straddles the areas of obstetrics and surgery, I provide a brief overview of writings in both fields before the fourteenth century. This material provides the background for an explanation of the changes that took place in the fourteenth and fifteenth centuries, when medical literature paid increasing attention to the operation. The laicization of surgery and the emergence of dissections in an academic setting were two important preconditions for the development of ideas on Caesarean section. (The brief overview of ideas prevalent in obstetrics and surgery at the time will be more useful to the general reader than to the specialist.) I then provide a survey and analyses of medical texts on Caesareans and of the practices and ideologies they represent from 1305 to the seventeenth century; the chapter ends with a detailed examination of the texts of François Rousset, an ardent proponent of Caesareans on living women in the late sixteenth century, and of his opponents. The controversies he was embroiled in reveal some of the ideological underpinnings of Renaissance medicine. Rousset's optimism regarding the survival of both mother and child in Caesarean births was not shared by his colleagues and did not survive him. Only now, in the twentieth century, has medicine fulfilled what Rousset hoped for: routine Caesareans in which both mother and child survive.

In Chapter 2, I examine the place of the iconographic tradition of Caesarean birth in the history of medical illustration. Medical illustrations were not confined to medical manuscripts. They often appeared in the Bible and in some romances, epics, and historical texts that featured medical scenes. In this context, I analyze the conditions of the production of such images and define the relationship between text and image, something that has not always been done for the study of medical iconography. The most important result of my iconographic study is the recognition of the displacement of female practitioners in the performance of Caesarean sections.

The explanations for this displacement offered in Chapter 3 center on the professionalization of medicine and on accusations of witchcraft leveled against midwives. Caesarean birth proves to be a key element in the transformations of fifteenth- and sixteenth-century German midwifery statutes: it is here that midwives first begin to lose control over one important part of childbirth. Some of the material in this chapter is not directly related to Caesarean birth but is necessary in order to define the areas of competency of medieval and Renaissance midwives as well as the criticism and accusations they were subjected to. Hand in hand with the efforts of the (male) medical establishment to marginalize women in all areas of the healing professions went attempts by the religious authorities to limit and discredit the activities of midwives. If midwives had concentrated exclusively on obstetrics their fate may have been different. But their knowledge in the areas of contraception and abortion made them dangerous; for many of them this meant demotion, persecution, and eventual death. In this context, regulations surrounding Caesarean birth (statutes of midwifery; canons of several church councils) complement and alter some of the ideas expressed in the classic studies of witchcraft.

The superstitions attached to midwifery led not only to the displacement of female practitioners but also to all sorts of fables and miracle stories, often involving Caesarean birth. Some of these will be examined in Chapter 4, where saintly and satanic obstetricians are engaged in the performance of Caesarean sections. Here the duality of Caesarean birth—and of its unnaturalness—becomes especially clear. While saints and the Virgin use the Caesarean operation to bring salvation to suffering women, devils (in various forms) are responsible for the Caesarean delivery of the Antichrist: a bizarre culmination in medieval thinking about Caesarean birth.

The Appendix deals with the origin of the term "Caesarean section" and concentrates on the learned tradition responsible for many (often erroneous) ideas about the operation that persist to this day. It illustrates the interplay (frequently based on false etymologies) between legendary and medical material, which produced an intricate pattern of beliefs and explanations centering on Caesarean birth. The most important result of the play of associations and etymologies was the belief that Julius Caesar was born by Caesarean section. In the Appendix, I trace the details of the gradual entrenchment of this idea in the medieval imagination and, at the same time, show how the learned and the popular spheres interacted in the creation of legends and etymologies.

Caesarean birth provides both a focal point and a point of departure for an exploration of medieval and Renaissance culture. Medical, legal, religious, and artistic problems as well as issues related to gender roles crystallize around the performance of Caesarean section. Many of these issues have been studied separately, but the whole question has never been addressed.[10] Because Caesarean birth was often surrounded by extreme conditions it was thought and written about differently from normal childbirth. This difference encourages an emphasis on the role of Caesarean birth as a cultural—rather than as a purely medical—phenomenon. While a similar emphasis could, and should, be claimed for normal childbirth, the special nature of Caesarean birth opens up some new and unexpected vistas into the lives and thoughts of medieval and Renaissance women and men.

I CAESAREAN BIRTH
IN MEDICAL THOUGHT

Caesarean birth had a place in medieval culture before it began to interest learned physicians. Medieval scholars interested in the ancient Romans and in the intricate problems of etymology occupied themselves with the question of the origin of Julius Caesar's name and whether he was born by Caesarean section; in addition, legends and miracles concerning Caesarean birth became part of the popular imagination.[1] Since the medieval ideas on Caesarean birth inherited from antiquity came from nonmedical sources, the operation did not appear in the canon of medical texts used by medieval physicians. It was not until the early fourteenth century that remarks on postmortem Caesarean sections began to emerge in medical treatises.

PREGNANCY, CHILDBIRTH, AND OBSTETRICS

She twisted and turned and writhed, this way, that way, to and fro, and continued so until, with much labour she bore a little son. But see, it lived, and she lay dead.[2]

> Madame saincte Marguerite,
> digne vierge de Dieu eslite,
> qui Dieu servis dés ta jeunesse,
> plaine de grace et de sagesse,
> qui pour l'amour de Nostre Sire
> souffris maint grant et grief martire,
> qui le dragon parmi fendis

et du tirant te deffendis,
qui vainquis l'ennemy d'enfer,
enchartree et liee en fer,
qui a Dieu feiz mainte requeste
quant on te voult couper la teste,
et par especial que femme
grosse d'enfant qui a toy, dame,
de cuer devot retourneroit,
et humblement te requerroit,
que Dieu de peril la gardast
et luy aider point ne tardast,
si te prie, vierge honoree,
noble martire et bieneuree,
par ta benoiste passion,
par ta sainte peticion,
que Dieu vueilles pour moy prier
et doulcement luy supplier
que par pitié il me conforte
es douleurs qu'i fault que je porte,
et sans peril d'ame et de corps
face mon enfant yssir hors
sain et sauf, si que je le voye
baptizé a bien et a joye.
Et se de vivre il a espace,
luy ottroye s'amour et sa grace,
par quoy si sainctement le serve
que la gloire des cieulx desserve.
Et aux autres, en cas semblable,
par toy soit doulx et favourable.

                    AMEN

([Medieval women in the throes of childbirth prayed to Saint Margaret:]
Madame, Saint Margaret, / worthy virgin, elected by God, / who served
God from her youth, / full of grace and wisdom, / who for the love of Our
Lord / suffered such a great and painful martyrdom, / who cut the dragon
in half / and defended yourself against the tyrant, / who vanquished the
enemy from hell / who was imprisoned and bound with iron, / who made
many a request to God / when they wanted to cut off your head, / and
especially when a woman / big with child who turns her devout heart
towards you / and humbly begs you / that God may save her from peril, /
and may not delay His help to her, / this is when I pray to you honored
virgin / noble and blessed martyr / through your blessed passion, / through
your saintly petition / may you pray to God for me / and sweetly ask Him /
that He may comfort me through His pity / in the pain which I have to
undergo / and that He—without danger to soul or body—make my child
come out / safe and sound, so that I can see him / baptized joyously. / And

so that he has room to live / may He give him His love and His Grace / for which he will serve Him in such a saintly way / that he may deserve the glory of the heavens. / And to others, in similar cases, through you, be sweet and favorable. Amen.)[3]

A fifteen-year old woman gives birth to a dead baby girl. Despite the devoted help of her chambermaid and a neighbor, after the birth she loses all sensation in her body below the waist. Burning candles and glowing coals are applied to her feet to test the insensitivity of her body—to no avail. For one and a half years no change in her condition occurs. It is only when she hears of the miracles that are happening at the tomb of Saint Louis (whose bones had been translated on that very day [May 22, 1281] to Saint Denis) that she envisions a possible cure for her ailment. She promises to attend mass every year at his anniversary, not to work on that day, and to become his pilgrim. After she touches the tomb and then the sick parts of her body, she lies down beside the tomb. Nine days later after having performed this ritual daily she feels how the bones in her body start banging together and on the tenth day she regains feeling in the lower part of her body. At the inquiry during Saint Louis's canonization trial her case is examined and witnesses state that she is still healthy (May 1282).

The first example above is Gottfried von Strassburg's early thirteenth-century description of Tristan's birth. Blancheflor, Tristan's mother, weakened through grief over the recent slaying of her husband, Riwalin, dies while giving birth. This scene undoubtedly reproduces many a medieval birth. Although medieval midwives were aware that emotional stress could result in difficult labor, they had few resources at their disposal that would allow them to prevent the tragic results of such complications.

The second example evokes Saint Margaret. Her story tells how she refused the Roman prefect Olibrius and rather than give up her virginity submitted to hideous tortures. She was then imprisoned and attacked in her prison by a terrifying dragon. When the monster did not manage to devour her, Olibrius finally had her burned with flaming torches and submerged in tubs of water. But she remained unharmed, and the crowd watching her began to be converted. Olibrius then decided to have her beheaded, and a moment before her death she prayed to God not only for herself and her executioners but also for any woman in labor: if the woman addressed herself to Saint Margaret for help the birth would have a happy outcome. A voice from heaven promised Margaret that her prayers would be fulfilled, and she went to her death reassured.

Saint Margaret's story was extraordinarily popular in the Middle Ages (it was included in Jacobus of Voragine's *Golden Legend*), but it is not obvious at first sight which elements in her life predestined her to become the patroness of women in labor. The mixture of ideals of virginity and extreme violence in her story parallels that in the lives of many other virgin martyrs who were raped, mutilated, or forced to enter bordellos before their execution. What distinguishes Saint Margaret's story is the presence and function of the dragon. In different versions of the legend Saint Margaret either avoids being swallowed by the dragon or emerges unharmed from its belly. Given the sexual connotations of the dragon—the Antichrist is often called a lascivious dragon and seducer, for example—and the beliefs that the dragon-viper gives birth by splitting open (the violent and deadly consequences of sexual activity, as Rabanus Maurus pointed out),[4] Saint Margaret's martyrdom evokes both sexual violence and the pains of childbirth, and it is perhaps for this reason that she offered a prayer for women in labor before her death. Birth, in an age before systematized contraception, was the natural consequence of sexual relations and, for some women at least, must have seemed to be a punishment for the pleasure they experienced during conception.[5] The violence connected with Saint Margaret's death must have recalled, for many medieval women, the violence they had experienced, either themselves or as witnesses, during childbirth.

The idealization of virginity and the consequent rejection of sexual pleasure, so prevalent in medieval art and theological writings, have their roots in antiquity. Philo of Alexandria (first century A.D.) exalted virginity as a way for women to approach the male level of rationality.[6] A few centuries later, Saint Jerome (340–420) confirmed this idea when he wrote that "as long as woman is for birth and children, she is different from man as body is from soul. But if she wishes to serve Christ more than the world, she will cease to be a woman and will be called a man."[7] And almost eleven centuries after Jerome, when the chancellor of the University of Paris wanted to bestow praise on Christine de Pizan he called her "distinguished woman, manly female" (*insignis femina, virilis femina*).[8]

It would be simplistic to see only male oppression and arrogance in this type of statement. As Margaret Miles states with regard to the depiction of women in fourteenth-century Tuscan painting: "The idealization of the virginal woman . . . may have symbolized to medieval women freedom from the burden of frequent childbearing and nursing in an age in which these natural processes were highly dangerous." Idealizing virginity may thus have helped women to master the "brutish" aspect of their biologically determined lives.[9]

We can now understand better why the Virgin Mary and Saint Margaret were invoked during childbirth. One gave birth without encountering any of the physical suffering related to it; the other sacrificed her life for her virginity but before her death had to undergo torments not unlike those experienced during childbirth. Through her ability to sympathize with tormented women she became their ideal intercessor.

The third example, the case history of a young medieval woman, is the third miracle in the collection of the *Miracles de Saint Louis,* by Guillaume de Saint-Pathus. It dramatizes the aftermath of a dead birth as a precarious condition for a woman. The symptoms, a type of paralysis (possibly of hysterical origin) resulting in a partial depersonalization, help the woman deny the existence of that part of her body connected with sex and reproduction. It is remarkable that neither the account of the cure nor the final testimony a year later even mentions the possibility of her having more children; nor does the husband appear. This absence is very telling for, as we will see later, medieval birth was entirely in the hands of women. The young woman's symptoms vanished, but the underlying causes—sexuality represented by the absent husband who could have caused another birth—continue to be denied and passed over in silence.

From these three examples medieval birth emerges with all its frightening and often fatal consequences. Where could medieval women find help and comfort in their trials? Before turning to some concrete examples let us briefly examine attitudes toward pregnancy and childhood (necessarily related to those toward motherhood) and what we can know about them in the Middle Ages in order to understand the feelings with which pregnant women and midwives approached the critical moment of childbirth.

Only one passage from the New Testament puts some value on childbearing: "Yet woman will be saved through bearing children, if she continues in faith and love and holiness, with modesty" (1 Tim. 2:15). We should not forget the context of this passage, however, which emphasizes women's duty to be submissive to men, their guilt as descendants of Eve, as well as the interdiction "I permit no woman to teach" (verse 12). Procreation here is seen as a way of salvation, albeit an inferior one. Even the command of Genesis "Be fruitful and multiply" was not generally interpreted, in the medieval period, as expressing a positive attitude toward childbirth. Not bodily reproduction but spiritual advancement was the real meaning of this command, according to Saint Thomas Aquinas (1225–74).[10] In general, the church's attitude toward marriage, sexuality, and pregnancy was negative.[11] There were some notable exceptions, such as Duns Scotus, who seems to have favored "limitless procreation" in order to restore the city of supernatural citizens in human nature.[12] But even here children are seen in a spiritual context and not as a value in themselves.

The teachings of the church do not always directly reflect contemporary reality, of course. It would be absurd to say that in the Middle Ages no one enjoyed sex and that parents did not want and love their children. Nevertheless, church teachings posit an ideal that Christians are urged to pursue. And, as Vern Bullough points out, "Church sexual ideals remained much the same at the end of the Middle Ages as they were at the beginning. Although . . . Church officials dealt with the world as they found it, the ascetic ideal still dominated, and *at best,* sexual activity was only to be tolerated providing it resulted in procreation."[13] Although childlessness may have serious consequences for noble families, such as disputes over inheritance and succession rights,[14] the general spiritual climate of the age did not favor ideas on childbearing as an important social function. In the hierarchy of medieval values, then, procreation and sex ranked extremely low. Thus, even outside of clerical writings, it is hard to come by positive remarks—or any definite remarks, for that matter—on medieval women as mothers.

Whereas many texts, legal and canonical as well as literary, discuss women's rights and duties as wives, they strangely neglect women's role as mothers.[15] Historians of the family have found several explanations for this scarcity of evidence. According to Philippe Ariès, children had no special place in medieval society.[16] Emotional attachments to children were not encouraged because of the high infant mortality; even Montaigne, in the sixteenth century, acknowledged that he lost "two or three" children in their infancy—not without regret, it is true, but not with too much *fascherie* (worry) either.[17]

One of the few literary texts that deal with childbirth is the fifteenth-century misogynistic treatise *Les quinze joies de mariage.* The eighth "joy" of marriage is that of childbirth: it gives a woman the opportunity to play sick and to assemble all her gossiping companions (*commères*) in the house who have nothing better to do than squander the poor husband's belongings.[18] The situation caricatured here reflects contemporary customs surrounding childbirth. Adrian Wilson has analyzed the importance of this ritual in anthropological terms. The sequence of separation, transition, and reincorporation (represented by the rite of churching) "conforms closely to the classical description of 'rites of passage' developed by Arnold van Gennep."[19] The "gossips," or "god-siblings," are an important part of the ritual: they prepare the lying-in room, provide nourishment for the attendants, and assure the sequestration of the mother. *Les quinze joies* provides a different and bitter view of this almost sacred ritual.

According to Ariès, the family as such (as opposed to the concept of lineage) had no emotional reality and consequently did not inspire poets and artists.[20] This view has been challenged recently in the work of Weinstein and Bell, who argue for "a close-knit, affective family, in which children were caringly treated on their own terms while being prepared for adulthood."[21] Weinstein and Bell, of course, deal with the childhood of saints whose families are depicted mostly in the vitae of these saints or in documents related to their canonization. The circumstances of these lives were extraordinary, and it was one of the goals of hagiography to emphasize this extraordinariness. Authors of vitae, even more than those of other medieval narrative genres, worked with topoi of which "the saint's family and his or her relationship to it" was certainly an important one. But there is a great variety in the families' reactions to their children's budding sainthood, and while these scenes are probably not a wholly realistic reflection of medieval family life, they nevertheless allow for some rare glimpses into the relationships between parents and children. Here, women as mothers, caring yet often skeptical when faced with their children's frequently peculiar behavior, make some of their rare and moving appearances in medieval texts.

Many medieval mothers were, like mothers at all periods in history, negligent in the care of their children. Accidental deaths of infants must have been quite common, as one can gather from a canon of the Council of Canterbury (1236) that urges priests to exhort mothers (every single Sunday) not to sleep in the same bed with their infants because they might accidentally smother them; also, infants were not to be left near fire or water without a guardian.[22] Accidents like these are described in miracle collections such as the *Miracles de Saint Louis*. The first miracle, for example, tells of a three-and-a-half-year-old girl who, while playing at a stream, dips her little bucket too far into the water. She loses her balance, falls into the stream, and is thought to have drowned. Friends of the parents retrieve the dead girl and try to revive her. When all their efforts fail, the parents invoke the aid of Saint Louis by promising him the weight of the girl in rye. At the end of the day, the little girl miraculously returns to life.

Miracle collections are a promising and as yet virtually untapped source of information on family relationships and attitudes toward children. In addition to the story just mentioned, there are many moving examples of parents who go to great lengths to procure help for their sick children. Mothers, fathers, and other family members take turns in spending time with the sick child, going through the rituals at Saint Louis's tomb but constantly worrying about the children they left at home. How realistic are these scenes? In a sense, the personnel for these testimonies is preselected: the parents in these accounts are by definition "good parents" because they took extraordinary trouble in seeking help for their children, however negligent they may have been earlier. Good parents and loving families clearly existed, but they were not a topic chosen by many medieval writers.

Aside from hagiography and miracle collections the literature of the time gives almost no place to mothers—or fathers for that matter— except to dramatize the tragic birth of a hero, as in the passage quoted at the beginning of this chapter, or to depict families in connection with the creation and perpetuation of a lineage.

For medieval saints, families were often seen as obstacles to spiritual salvation. The mystic Angela of Foligno, for example, considered the death of her entire family (including her mother) not only a deliverance from earthly ties but an answer to her prayers.[23] In his *Miroir de mariage* the poet Eustache Deschamps lists more practical reasons for despising children: in infancy they create only noise, bad smells, trouble, and worry; they have to be fed and clothed; their lives are constantly at risk and should they manage to reach adulthood they could very well end up in prison. Positive attitudes toward childhood are hard to come by whether we look in clerical or secular writings. No wonder, then, that attitudes toward pregnancy were hardly more positive. Spiritually inferior and medically at great risk, the pregnant woman had little to look forward to. As Myra Leifer has pointed out, cultural and social pressures play an important role in pregnancy.[24] These pressures were mostly negative in the Middle Ages and thus added to the burden any pregnancy, even the most desired, represented in a woman's life. From the many accounts of seventeenth- and eighteenth-century childbirth studied by Mireille Laget, a conclusion emerges that also holds true for the Middle Ages: "the woman appears traumatized by previous confinements or by the many stories she has heard."[25] The only people whom the pregnant medieval woman could turn to (except to her patron saint) and who could sympathize with her were other women.

At most births in the Middle Ages only women were present. An exception to this rule was royal birth. We know, for example, that in 1101, at the birth of her first child, Queen Matilda, the wife of the English king Henry I, was assisted by two Italian physicians, a layman named Grimbald and the abbot of Abingdon, Faritius.[26] Whether they assisted with the actual birth is not quite clear. They may just have been observers or in charge of the astrological speculations that accompanied every important birth. In any case, Matilda, unlike the unfortunate Blancheflor who did not survive the birth of her son Tristan, went on to have two more children but lost this first son while he was still an infant. Generally, however, birth belonged to the domain of daily life and was, if all went well, a nonmedical process. As indicated in the scene of the *Les quinze joies,* mothers, grandmothers, and neighbors would be present in addition to the midwife, who was a lay practitioner and often a person in possession of folk wisdom.

Certainly up to the fifteenth century being a midwife was not a profession; it was an activity, learned by apprenticeship, that involved as much psychological as physical assistance during and after the birth.[27]

Childbirth had, of course, been treated in the classical corpus of medical texts, the Hippocratic and the Galenic. However, obstetrical material was not presented as a separate handbook, which could have been of use to midwives, for example. It was embedded in the theoretical discourse on conception, menstruation, and pregnancy, largely concerned with humoral theories, which governed every aspect of a human's well-being.

Several texts included speculations on what triggered the actual birth. The Hippocratics, for example, believed that, alarmed by the lack of food, the fetus would begin the birth process by its own initiative,[28] while Galen introduced the concepts of the *vis propultrix* and the *vis expultrix* as the two forces that govern the two phases of birth. Other areas of concern were the positions of the fetus (only head first was considered natural) and how to remove a dead fetus (by violent shaking or with surgical instruments).

It was not until the appearance of Soranus of Ephesos's *Gynecology* (second century A.D.) that questions of female physiology, pregnancy, and birth were treated separately. Portions of his text survive only in later translations, that of Caelius Aurelianus (fifth century) and Moschion (sixth century). Soranus evidently had great confidence in the capacities of midwives, and he devotes twenty-eight chapters in his second book to pregnancy, childbirth, and the treatment and possible diseases of the newborn.

Soranus begins by describing the signs announcing the imminent birth and then specifies how a room should be prepared for a woman's labor: warm water, sponges, warm fomentations for the alleviation of pain, bandages (for swaddling), and "things to smell to revive the laboring woman" should be present.[29] He describes the birth stool in great detail, specifying the size of the cut-outs, the shape of the back and so on.[30] His instructions for the actual birth show great attention to the feelings of the woman in labor: the midwife should do nothing that may seem undignified or upsetting to the future mother. The positions indicated for the midwife and the helpers (one holding the woman from the back, the others at her sides) became a standard for obstetrical illustrations, as we will see in Chapter 2. The birth itself requires care and patience on the part of the midwife, who must beware of rupturing the perineum. The woman herself has to participate actively in the birth; Soranus makes it clear that mental attitudes play a role in this essentially physiological process. Once the child is born the "majority of women practising midwifery" approve of cutting the umbilical cord with glass, a reed, or other sharp objects but not with a knife. Here Soranus comments: "cutting with iron is deemed of ill omen. This is absolutely ridiculous, [for] crying itself is of ill omen, and yet it is with this that the child begins its life." Thus it is better to "be less superstitious and cut the navel cord with a knife."[31] Advice on cleansing, swaddling, and feeding the infant follows. Soranus is very explicit on how to select a wet nurse and what kind of regimen the nurse should follow in order to have healthy milk.[32] Bathing (not too often so as not to soften the newborn) and massaging the newborn have the purpose of giving it the correct shape. For example, holding the child upside down will untangle the vertebrae.[33] Soranus spends several pages on detailed instructions on how to mold the child, an indication of how "unfinished" and malleable the newborn was considered to be. Walking, weaning and teething, tonsillitis, itching, and flux of the bowels are the subjects that close book 2.

Difficult birth is treated in book 4. The causes are divided into those relating to the mother and those relating to the infant.[34] A large part of the text is devoted to detailed instructions (addressed to midwives) for version of the unborn in case of unnatural presentation. Although Soranus advises great delicacy and caution for any internal version, it is clear that his advice could rarely be applied competently: most midwives did not have the skills necessary for the maneuvers of a successful version; and since no hygienic precautions were taken, the intervention supposed to assure the mother's salvation often brought about her death.

The advice on version of the unborn reappears in later medical texts, notably in the *De passionibus mulierum,* now known as *Cum auctor,* a text for centuries wrongly attributed to so-called Trotula, or Trota, presumably a twelfth-century female physician from Salerno.[35] In a Middle English version of this text no fewer than sixteen ways of unnatural presentation are described with "advice on how they are to be rectified."[36] While Soranus did not subscribe to some of the rather questionable methods proposed by some medical writers (for example, the violent shaking of pregnant women to induce the birth [often of a dead child]), even he called for desperate measures in the case of a permanently stalled birth: "If the fetus does not respond to manual traction, because of its size, or death, or impaction in any manner whatsoever, one must proceed to more forceful methods, those of extraction by hooks and embryotomy. For even if one loses the infant, it is still necessary to take care of the mother."[37] Again, Soranus goes into great detail concerning the procedures of extraction by hooks and embryotomy where it finally made no difference whether the fetus was dead or still alive. The methods of fragmenting a fetus are described soberly: the first and foremost concern was to save the mother. For Soranus, Caesarean section does not exist as an option for terminating a protracted birth.

In the *Trotula* translated by Mason-Hohl, the only methods recommended for removing a dead fetus are induced sneezing, and if this does not work, "let the patient be placed in a linen cloth stretched by four men at the four corners with the patient's head somewhat elevated and she will give birth immediately, God favoring her."[38] The contrast with Soranus's text is striking. He devotes two extensive chapters to the removal of a dead (or impacted) fetus; the treatment in this popular medieval text is more than scanty.

Soranus's *Gynecology* contained much medical information and sensitive advice regarding childbirth. But although his text and its translations were transmitted to medieval Europe, it is not clear whether midwives could actually profit from these texts. Given the low rate of female literacy, at least up to the fifteenth century, it is likely that midwives, if they knew the texts at all, could have heard of them only indirectly. Probably knowledge of Soranus's tradition was largely confined to the learned sphere.[39]

The texts of Hippocrates, Galen, Avicenna, and others (as well as the many commentaries on them) became part of the university curriculum and were studied by physicians whose interest in practical medicine was limited and in obstetrics, almost nonexistent.[40]

But purely medical texts were not the only source for advice on childbirth. Bartholomeus Anglicus, the thirteenth-century encyclopedist, described the function of the midwife as follows: "The midwife is a woman who possesses the art of helping a woman in childbirth so that the birth goes easier and the infant is not endangered."[41] While Bartholomeus had dealt with theories of conception (based on Avicenna) in book 5 of his treatise and turned to diseases in book 7, the remarks on midwives, wet nurses, and the care of the newborn infant are part of book 6, "De etatibus hominis" (Of the ages of man), which deals with a man's household and his family. Childbirth is thus presented in a nonmedical context.

As in many other parts of his book, Bartholomeus here relies heavily on ancient authorities while at the same time displaying a gift for the observation and description of contemporary daily life. Thus his remarks regarding the care of the newborn owe much to such writers as Constantinus Africanus, the famous eleventh-century translator of Arabic medical texts, but they probably also reflect what medieval midwives were expected to do. This included the cutting and tying up of the umbilical cord, and the washing of the infant, who was then dried in the sun or in front of a fire. Ointments were applied to the child's body and its palate and gums were rubbed with honey. Finally the baby was wrapped in soft cloths, often tightly wrapped swaddling clothes, as one can see in manuscript illuminations (for example, figs. 1 and 2). In accordance with Galenic theories, the newborn was seen as moist and soft and thus needed to be constricted in its movements.[42] While today it is believed that swaddling actually comforts the newborn, Salvat suggests (without any direct evidence, however) that in the Middle Ages this practice may have been symbolic of the imprisonment by sin that the infant is subject to at the moment of its birth—not exactly a consoling thought for the new mother, who had just gone through the ordeal of labor.[43]

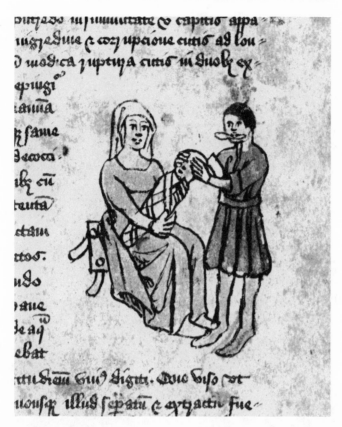

1. A head operation (John of Arderne, *Speculum flebotomiae*, University of Glasgow Library, MS Hunter 112, fol. 94r)

Bartholomeus's placing of childbirth in the chapter on the ages of man signals how childbirth was perceived in the Middle Ages. Despite the myriad medical writings on the subject, birth was still in the hands of midwives and consequently a nonmedicalized procedure, a part of daily life ruled by empiricism and not in the domain of the physician, a part that had not yet been embraced by what Foucault terms "le regard médical."[44] As for Caesarean sections, we can draw a preliminary conclusion at this point: while some of the ancient authorities mention surgical instruments in the context of embryotomy (the removal of a dead fetus in parts), none of them deals with surgical delivery as such.

The preceding paragraphs are, of course, not an exhaustive treatment of medieval birth or of the ideas on childbirth by medical writers. They

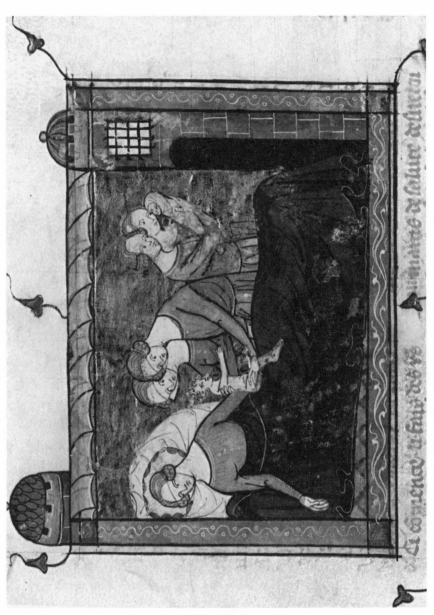

2. The birth of Julius Caesar (*Les Faits des Romains*, Paris, B.N. f. fr. 251, fol. 21sr)

serve only to recreate, at least in part, the atmosphere, attitudes, and fears that must have attended any birth in the medieval and Renaissance period when the physician's involvement in childbirth was mostly theoretical and midwives had no effective means at their disposal to ease the pain of childbirth or to avoid complications during deliveries that often spelled the death of the mother. Frequent stillbirths and miscarriages and a high mortality rate of infants added to the stress experienced by medieval women during pregnancy. Caesarean section, representing as it does violence and mutilation, epitomizes the dangers of medieval and Renaissance childbirth. In the popular imagination it belonged to the realm of legends and miracles, but for midwives it was an eventuality they had to be prepared for.

The earliest testimonies of Caesarean birth do not mention midwives because there the operation appears mostly in a legal context or in works dealing with etymology. The actual performance of the operation was not of primary concern to the earliest witnesses, some of which we will now consider.

EARLY TRADITIONS OF CAESAREAN BIRTH

The oldest presumed testimony of a Caesarean birth, from the second millennium B.C., appears in a cuneiform tablet from Mesopotamia, which contains a legal text dealing with the adoption of a small boy.[45] The child is described as one "who was pulled out from the womb." Although, of course, pulling is not cutting, a Caesarean section may be meant; since the use of forceps for the delivery of a living child was unknown until the early modern period, it is unlikely that a normal birth would be referred to in such terms.[46] In addition, "to pull the baby out" is exactly the term used to describe a Caesarean section in the marginal instructions to the illuminator in the manuscript Princeton Garrett 128 (fig. 3).[47] Most likely, then, this phrase refers to a Caesarean section.

The first explicit mention of Caesarean birth goes back to about 715 B.C., when the *lex regia* was proclaimed by the Roman king Numa Pompilius. The law stated that it was unlawful to bury an undelivered woman before the child had been cut out. Whoever broke this law caused a living being to die together with the pregnant woman.[48] The *lex regia* was transmitted by the sixth-century Byzantine emperor Justinian I through his *Digesta,* a compilation of legal texts.[49] From the existence of

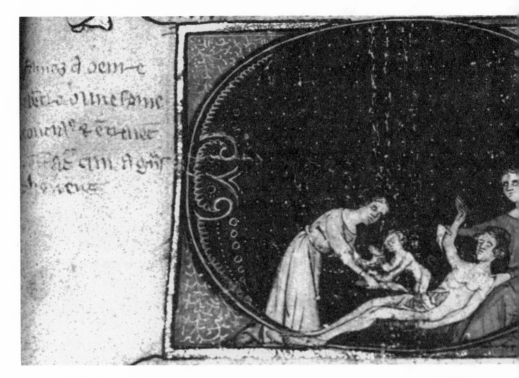

3. The birth of Julius Caesar (*Les Faits des Romains*, Princeton University Library, MS Garrett 128, fol. 144r)

this law one can conclude that Caesarean sections were performed post-mortem in order to save the child. Unfortunately neither the indication for a Caesarean nor possible techniques were mentioned.

Another early testimony can be found in the writings of the Indian doctor Sûsruta, who lived sometime between the fifth century B.C. and the second century A.D. In chapter 8 of his *Nidânasthâna* he urges a Caesarean in case the mother dies during birth and movements of the child can still be detected. The operation has to be done quickly, he adds, for a delay could cause the death of the child.[50] Other Indian medical writers in the early Middle Ages repeat this advice.

Early Jewish culture also seems to have known of Caesarean birth. A passage from the Mishna, which contains texts from the third century B.C. to about the third century A.D., states that "in the case of twins, neither the first child which shall be brought into the world by the cut in the abdomen, nor the second can receive rights of primogeniture, either

as regards the office of priest, or succession to property."[51] Was a Caesarean ever practiced on living women in this early period? Jeffrey Boss is
convinced that Caesareans with maternal survival were quite common in
the Jewish tradition, but even he has to admit that "the mother's recovery
after caesarean section is implicit rather than explicit in the relevant
passages."[52] From the following passage in the Nidda, an appendix to the
Talmud, it has often been concluded that Jewish culture knew and
practiced this operation on living women: "It is not necessary for women
to observe the days of purification, after removal of a child through the
parieties of the abdomen."[53] The medieval commentator, physician, and
author of medical texts Maimonides (1135–1204) advised that an incision
should be made in the woman's side and that she should in this way be
delivered of her child.[54] It is not clear whether in this case the survival of
the woman was assumed. The mention of the dispensation from purification would suggest that it was; but possibly this passage is of a purely
theoretical nature, which would correspond to a tendency in Jewish
commentaries to provide for even the most unlikely cases. For the time
being, then, the question of maternal survival of Caesareans in the ancient Jewish world has to be left unresolved.

The next witness to Caesarean birth, Pliny the Elder (A.D. 23–79),
makes much of the auspiciousness of Caesarean birth when he discusses
the term *caesones* in his *Natural History* (7.9), but he supplies no medical
information. (Still, his text is important for the history of the term
"Caesarean section"; see Appendix.)

In Greek and Byzantine medical writings no mention is made of the
operation.[55] In the Islamic world, the tenth-century chronicler al-Bīrūnī
mentioned the operation in the context of the birth of Julius Caesar: an
illustration in a fourteenth-century manuscript of his *Chronology of Ancient Nations* shows a group of bearded men surrounding an obviously
dead woman just delivered by Caesarean. Peter Soucek suggests that this
illustration was based on a medical handbook (although he does not say
which one).[56] Several Arabic writers indicated the possibility of surgical
intervention during birth with instructions for midwives or surgeons,
but they do not mention Caesarean section.[57] From the indications
supplied by Manfred Ullmann one can conclude that certain operations,
such as the removal of a woman's bladder stones, were performed by
midwives (or "chaste" surgeons) under the supervision of a physician.[58]
Later, Western medical writers, such as François Rousset, likened the
operation for bladder stones (in terms of surgical technique) to the

Caesarean operation, but in the Arabic tradition there is unfortunately no evidence of such a parallel; it would give us some insight into whether and how the operation was performed.

How, then, did the Caesarean section become part of medicine and how does it fit into the medieval medical canon? And how did midwives eventually know of and learn about the operation?

We find no remarks on Caesarean sections performed post-mortem in the European tradition before the early fourteenth century. Since in this operation the mother's death was presupposed and the fetus's death almost certain, it is likely that the Caesarean section was initially not considered a medical procedure and consequently had no place in the canonical works of school medicine. If it was part of medicine at all, it belonged to the realm of surgery rather than obstetrics, although in its early stages the operation was performed mostly by midwives. There is no one explanation for the entry of Caesarean section into medical works; rather, the preconditions must be sought in many areas.

SURGERY, CAESAREAN BIRTH, AND DISSECTION BEFORE 1300

Although a few Caesarean births are mentioned in various early medieval texts, the operation as a medical procedure is not known to appear in medical writings prior to Bernard of Gordon, a Montpellier physician, who mentions it in book 7 of his compendium *Practica sive lilium medicinae* (1305). I would suggest that a combination of factors led to the inclusion of the operation in learned treatises: the laicization of surgery; the increasingly explicit directions for Caesareans issued by various church councils; the new definitions of areas of professional competency regarding physicians and surgeons; and finally the performance of autopsies and dissections, which started in the thirteenth century.

In the early Middle Ages medicine was in the hands of the clergy. Both monks and nuns could act as physicians, and nuns could take over the office of midwife in the community to which the convent was attached.[59] Hildegard of Bingen is well-known as a woman belonging to a religious order who was knowledgeable about medicine and wrote several medical books.[60] Often nuns had to act as physicians and surgeons out of sheer necessity, to staff hospices and hospitals, for example. Surgery at this time consisted mostly in bloodletting and the treatment of wounds.[61]

The laicization of surgery began in the twelfth century when the church forbade its clergy to perform procedures that involved the shedding of blood. At its origin this interdiction had nothing to do with the church's "abhorrence of blood." The first interdictions against the practice of medicine and law on the part of the clergy had different and more general motivations. Canon number 5 of the Council of Clermont in 1130, canon 6 of the Council of Rheims in 1131, and canon 9 of the Second Lateran Council in 1139 all state that "monks and canons regular are not to study jurisprudence and medicine for personal gain."[62] Thus monks and canons regular (that is, members of the regular clergy) were excluded from the practice of these two professions because through them they might fall into the sins of avarice and cupidity and forget their true vocation: to serve God and save souls.[63] At the Council of Tours in 1163, Pope Alexander III warned the clergy against entanglement in the affairs of this world.[64] The canon "Ecclesia abhorret a sanguine" (The church abhors blood) often attributed to the Council of Tours is a literary fiction that proved surprisingly tenacious despite Charles H. Talbot's observation that the phrase "owes its existence to Quesnay, the uncritical historian of the Faculty of Surgeons at Paris, who in 1774, citing a passage from Pasquier's *Recherches de la France* ["et comme l'église n'abhorre rien tant que le sang"] translated it into Latin and put it into italics."[65] No earlier source for this sentence can be found.[66] Originally, then, the practice of medicine was proscribed only as part of a dangerous involvement in worldly affairs, especially if it was practiced for gain and not out of compassion.

In 1215, at the Fourth Lateran Council, those members of the secular clergy who had taken major orders (subdeacons, deacons, and priests) were included in a new interdiction against the practice of that part of surgery that involved cutting and burning (phlebotomy and cauterization). Even if these interdictions were not always observed, as Ernest Wickersheimer has shown, they were nevertheless responsible for the laicization of surgery and for the beginning of the power struggle between different groups of professionals.[67] We can now understand why the Caesarean operation, a medical procedure that consisted of "cutting" and that took place post-mortem, could not be part of clerical medicine and was initially left to midwives.

The church prescribed Caesareans primarily for the sake of baptizing the newborn child. It seems that the Parisian archbishop Odon de Sully (1196–1208) was the first church official to recommend a Caesarean if there was a chance that the child was still alive after the death of the mother: "Mortuae in partu scindantur, si infans credatur vivere; tamen si bene constiterit de morte earum" (Those who have died in childbirth should be cut open when the child is believed to be still alive; however, it has to be well established that they are dead).[68] The Council of Canterbury in 1236 stipulated that in case of the mother's death her body should be cut and the child extracted. The mother's mouth should be held open during this procedure. The same council urged women to confess themselves before they went into labor, and midwives were instructed to prepare water for a possible emergency baptism.[69] Thus the midwife had to be prepared for the eventuality of a fatal outcome of any birth she attended. She had to make quick decisions, for the eternal salvation of the infant was at stake.

How complex and problematic these decisions were can be seen from a text composed at the Council of Trèves in 1310: "Should a woman die during childbirth her body should be opened immediately and the child be baptized if it is still alive. If it is already dead it has to be buried outside of the cemetery. However, if one can assume that the child is already dead in its mother's body both of them should be buried in consecrated ground."[70] This passage has often been cited in order to underline the importance of the baptism of newborns. But it also points up the dilemma that a medieval midwife could find herself in. The salvation of the child, both physically and spiritually, depended exclusively on her. A mistake in her judgment could lead to the burial of the child in unconsecrated ground. The risk of the infant's spiritual damnation could be greatly lessened, it seems, if the question of its physical survival is treated as secondary, that is, if the midwife "decides" that the child is already dead before a Caesarean can be attempted. That midwives were deeply concerned with the newborn's salvation can be seen from the many accusations leveled against them for secretly baptizing stillborn children and burying them in consecrated ground.[71]

Another important decision confronted the midwife: should the mother ever be sacrificed for the sake of her child? Since baptism was of such paramount importance, the "hastened" death of the mother may have allowed the midwife to save an otherwise doomed child. Saint Thomas Aquinas in his teachings on baptism provides a clear answer to this question: " 'Evil should not be done that good may come,' according to St. Paul [Rom. 3:8]. Therefore one should not kill the mother in order to baptize the child; if, however, the child be still alive in the womb after the mother has died, the mother should be opened in order to baptize the child."[72] This opinion is reiterated in the sixteenth century by Saint Charles Borromeus.[73] Thus the choice indicated by Henry VIII, "Save the child by all means, for it is easier to get wives than children," was not the one recommended by such religious thinkers as Saint Thomas.[74] In fact, in the English translation of the text attributed to Trotula midwives were openly advised to kill the child rather than to risk the life of the mother: "whan the woman is feble and the chyld may noght comyn out, then it is better that the chylde be slayne than the moder of the child also dye."[75] Of course, the church was against abortion, but it seems that at least in the context of Caesarean birth the question of a *choice* between the mother's or the child's life never arose.

The midwife, then, deemed competent and even urged to be familiar with the rituals of baptism, stood at the borderline between different groups who contended for the salvation of the patient: the clergy, now unable to intervene surgically, and the lay surgeons, whose areas of competency grew not only through the new restrictions of clerical medicine but also, as we will see, because of new requirements concerning autopsies and dissections.

One area that has some bearing on the question of Caesarean birth is the conflict that seems to have existed between clerical and lay physicians about who was to be present at a person's deathbed. Whereas in earlier councils, such as the Council of Canterbury (1236), the sick were urged to call first a "physician of souls" (canon 34), later councils, such as the Council of Ravenna (1311), had somewhat more faith in the "physician of bodies," who is given at least one chance at saving the patient before a "doctor of souls" has to be called in: "We alert all doctors that they are not allowed to *return* to the patient before they have assured themselves that he has called a doctor of souls and has taken care of his spiritual salvation."[76] But after this first attempt, the hope for physical salvation had to give way to the hope for spiritual salvation. Thus science is given a chance, but faith has the last word.

It seems, then, that one of the results of the laicization of surgery was an increased presence of laymen at the moment of a person's death. A Caesarean, performed as it was post-mortem, could now interest surgeons. The operation began to move from the purely religious sphere

(religious, at least as far as the *motivation,* that is, baptism, was concerned) to a medical one. Although male surgeons did not perform the
operation at this point, it began to attract the attention of medical
writers, such as Bernard of Gordon.

In the century preceding Bernard some shifting had occurred in the
areas of competency assigned to physicians and surgeons. From a practical (not a theoretical) perspective the interests and the healing activities
of university-trained physicians had been rather limited. They consisted
largely in uroscopy, the taking of the pulse, the consultation of astrological charts, and the prescription of various herbal concoctions. Although
in the early Middle Ages bloodletting, or phlebotomy, had been the task
of the physician, in the later Middle Ages it and most other surgical
interventions were left to surgeons and barbers who learned their trade
through apprenticeship.[77] Thus the practical activities of physicians were
more restricted than they had been in earlier periods. Professional fields
had to be redefined, a process that led to a split between physicians and
surgeons.

In France, this split began in earnest after the emancipation of the
Faculty of Medicine at the University of Paris in 1272, when new rules
governing the issue of licenses went into effect.[78] Some twenty years later
the Italian surgeon Lanfranc of Milan (d. 1315) came to Paris to teach
among other subjects the surgical material then current at Bologna. He
deplored the rivalry between surgeons and physicians and pointed out
that a good practitioner should be well versed in surgery and medicine.[79]
Pouchelle suggests that Lanfranc's courses, given as they were at the Faculty of Medicine, may have caused physicians to fear even more for their
cherished domain of school medicine.[80] A surgeon was regarded as an in-
truder in the confines of the university of Paris; consequently, in the fourteenth century, Henri de Mondeville, although a surgeon of great fame,
was forced to teach outside of the university.[81] The surgeons, for their
part, showed the same disdain toward the barbers that the university-
trained doctors displayed toward the surgeons.[82] Thus those medical
treatises which showed a strong interest in surgery—and which began to
treat Caesarean sections—did not come from Paris but, rather, from
places like Montpellier, where surgery formed part of the school curriculum.

The division between the different professional groups was of course
not as radical as the various decrees to this effect would make it appear.

There were always individuals who did not conform to the strict rules desired by university-trained doctors. In general, a great discrepancy existed between medical theory and practice, but some medical practitioners managed to bridge this gap through their writings.[83] Even though close to 70 percent of French medical writings from the thirteenth to the fifteenth centuries were the work of university-trained physicians, two of the most interesting medical treatises of the fourteenth century were written by the surgeon-authors Henri de Mondeville and Guy de Chauliac (who were, however, among the last of their genre, as Pouchelle points out).[84]

Because medical compendia like Bernard of Gordon's contained a number of surgical elements from preceding centuries, we should also consider, however briefly, the tradition of surgical writing before the fourteenth century. In the twelfth century, an important compilation of surgical texts (mostly based on classical sources), now known as the *Bamberg Surgery,* had been assembled in Salerno; it was soon supplanted by Roger of Frugardi's text on surgery, especially important to surgeons in Bologna and to Guillelmus de Congenis of Montpellier.[85] Also in the twelfth century, Gerard of Cremona made available Arabic surgical treatises in Latin translations, which influenced the Italian surgeons Bruno da Longoburgo, Hugh of Lucca and his son Theodoric of Cervia, and William of Saliceto and his student Lanfranc of Milan.

Thus the thirteenth century produced a number of important surgical treatises that incorporated practical experience often gained on the battlefield. Lanfranc, for example, begins his treatise with extensive sections on different types of wounds and, with the exception of a few theoretical chapters, concentrates on the practices of bloodletting and cauterization and such matters as the treatment of cataracts, what to do about the swelling of limbs (apostemas), and the surgical removal of stones. The comprehensiveness of Lanfranc's treatise reminds us that surgery was, according to Dino del Garbo (a student of Taddeo Alderotti), one of the three important ways "of treating a sick body (the others were diet and medication.)"[86] The surgical aspects of obstetrics, such as embryotomy, which were very prominent in the Arabic tradition, had no place in a treatise like Lanfranc's.

Surgical treatises (originating mostly in Italy) left their mark on thirteenth-century medical compilations, such as Gilbertus Anglicus's *Compendium medicinae,* which contains several quotations of Roger of Parma's *Chirugia.*[87] The *Compendium,* based on Aristotelian principles and the ideas on the four humors, also features many recipes. Its subtitle (*Nondum medicis sed cyrurgicis utilissimum,* (Most useful not only for physicians but also for surgeons) underlines its usefulness for both professional groups. It begins with a treatise on fevers and then covers a large variety of diseases, beginning with those of the head and ending with diseases of the reproductive organs. Gilbertus concludes with remarks on such varied topics as leprosy and dog bites. In the tradition of medical *compendia* he deals with pregnancy and delivery, but it is interesting that he does not go into details of the surgical removal of a dead fetus, let alone Caesarean section. The only recommendations in this context are various fumigations and induced sneezing (fols. 306 and 307). The *Compendium*'s structure provided the model for Bernard of Gordon's *Lilium,* but Gilbertus's scanty treatment of obstetrical and gynecological questions cannot be compared with Bernard's extensive chapters on these subjects. Bernard does appear, then, for some areas at least, as an innovator. Before turning to Bernard's text let us briefly look at one more important factor that conditioned the medical milieu of the early fourteenth century: the history of dissection, which began in the late thirteenth century.

The teaching of anatomy required dissections, but before the late thirteenth century only animals were dissected. The observations made during these procedures were then applied, with modifications of course, to humans. Many misconceptions regarding human anatomy were thus created and perpetuated. This is not to say that once human cadavers were dissected these misconceptions disappeared: observation did not necessarily supersede received book learning.[88] Dissection was, rather, the "solemn illustration of the learning inherited from the ancients," especially Galen, whose texts were read as an accompaniment to the practical demonstration.[89] But dissection did allow for some new insights.[90] It also broke the taboo of opening up the human body.

In 1299 Pope Boniface VIII promulgated a bull that raised some questions on the admissibility of human dissection. It forbade the boiling of human cadavers in order to separate the flesh and the bones. Apparently this technique was used so that the bones of crusaders who died abroad could be repatriated and was seen by the pope as a violation of the integrity of the human body.[91] It seems that the church never expressed a clear opinion on the subject of anatomical dissection.[92] Thus the bull does not seem to prohibit dissection as such; its injunctions only preclude the study of skeletal anatomy.

It was toward the end of the thirteenth century that the first dissections were done in Bologna, an innovation "associated with the circle of Taddeo [Alderotti]" and the new requirements of academic medicine.[93] Even before Mondino de Luizzi, the author of the influential *Anatomia* (1316/17), began to conduct regular dissections as part of the university curriculum, Taddeo alluded to a dissection, stating that he could not solve a certain problem because he had been unable to examine the anatomy of a pregnant woman.[94] But, as Nancy Siraisi points out, it was only in response to the needs of a privileged and organized faculty of arts and sciences that regular dissections could take place.[95]

Dissections were conducted according to a certain ritual order, described by Guy de Chauliac in his *Grande chirurgie* (1363). Each successive stage was accompanied by a lecture: "the first on the digestive system, liver, and veins, . . . the second on the heart and arterial system, the third on the brain and nervous system, and the fourth on the extremities."[96] But dissections were not done frequently, even in Bologna. In France, regular dissections began to be performed in Montpellier in 1376 (despite a stipulation of 1340 that a dissection should take place every two years); the Faculty of Medicine in Paris waited until 1407 to perform its first dissection, which seems to have been more of an autopsy.[97]

In France, autopsies brought surgeons into contact with the judicial authorities as early as the beginning of the fourteenth century. The surgeon's reports are not very revealing, stating in one case that a certain butcher had indeed died from a fall into a well but without any visible wounds, or in another that a certain woman's head wound stemmed from an ax.[98] But we have to appreciate the efforts made at the turn from the thirteenth to the fourteenth century to base judgments on evidence obtained through the surgeons' first-hand observation, as inadequate as their expertise may appear to us today.

Through dissections and autopsies, then, the taboo of opening the human body was broken. These developments most likely contributed to Bernard of Gordon's decision to include remarks on Caesarean section in his *Lilium*. His is the first known Western text dealing with the operation, and thus he is a privileged witness for the textual developments of Caesarean birth. Then, in the fifteenth century, when it seemed that Caesarean birth could be wrested away from the realm of death, newly confident surgeons began to describe how they themselves performed the operation. The trend of medical optimism culminated in François Rousset's writings in the late sixteenth century, only to be obliterated by the subsequent generation of surgeons in the seventeenth.

THE TEXTUAL TRADITION OF
CAESAREAN BIRTH

Bernard of Gordon most likely spent his whole life in southwestern France. He probably studied and certainly taught at Montpellier in the late thirteenth and early fourteenth centuries.[99] The division between surgery and university medicine was not as pronounced in Montpellier as it was in Paris. Surgery was taught together with medicine and "practised by physicians."[100] Practical experience was required for licensing. As Demaitre has shown, even though the manual operations were left to surgeons, the *doctrina* of surgery formed part of the university education of physicians.[101] Arnold of Villanova, for example, accused his Parisian and northern colleagues of "too much absorption in book lelarning," a good indication that practical matters were of great importance in Montpellier.[102] In this context it makes sense that the two earliest texts that give a place—however small—to postmortem Caesarean birth should originate in a milieu that valued surgery and boasted a number of first-rate physicians, such as Bernard and Guy de Chauliac, who, in addition to their university education, showed an interest or had received excellent training in surgery. Although their texts were steeped in the works of the ancients (Guy's citations of ancient and contemporary authors go into the thousands) and medical astrology was a favorite topic, there is some evidence of first-hand observation and practical thinking. Thus Bernard emended ancient authorities on the basis of "reason and experience."[103] Like many other medical writers he frequently persuades his reader to accept certain findings as the results of personal experiments or deliberations while really relying on such works as Gilbertus Anglicus's *Compendium medicinae*.[104] But there are instances where Bernard clearly acknowledges learning something about certain remedies *per viam experimenti* from old wives (*a vetulis*).[105]

Bernard conceived his work as one of medical practice and explicitly named "the humble" as his target audience, that is, novice physicians and, most likely, surgeons.[106] Despite the importance accorded to surgery it was not a privileged method of treatment, for Bernard lists diet, regimen, medication, and surgery in descending order of preference.[107] A surgeon, for him, was a *restaurator* to whom one turned as a last resort. Caesarean section, although not a procedure of "restoration," certainly is in line with the idea of a last resort.

It is in Bernard's *Lilium,* then, that we find the first known mention, in Western medicine, of Caesarean birth.[108] At the end of book 7, chapter 15, "De regimine praegnantium," he cites Galen on the causes that initiate the birth: as a fruit falls from the tree so the fetus causes the rupture of the ligaments that hold it; they become fragile because of overextension and lack of nourishment. Immediately after these remarks, Bernard says that sometimes, even though the mother dies, the fetus may survive, at least for a certain time, through the air that still is in the mother's arteries. In that case, the mother's mouth should be opened and an incision should be made in her abdomen through which the child should be extracted. He also advises that the cervix be held open to assure the influx of air during the operation. The method is referred to as *artificium,* that is, an artificial means. Bernard does not given any clear indication of where the incision is supposed to be located. He closes his remarks with a reference to the birth of "the first of the Caesars."[109]

Given Bernard's other references to advice gathered from "old wives," one can speculate whether he learned about the operation from them. On the other hand, Bernard's reference to the legend of the birth of the "first of the Caesars" shows a familiarity with the learned tradition of the etymology of Caesar's name. But Pliny, the likely source for Bernard's reference, does not mention any medical details of the operation. In the learned textual tradition of medicine, as we saw above, Caesarean section was not mentioned. Consequently, the knowledge of the operation most likely has another origin, probably hearsay combined with some theoretical thoughts based on what was known about surgery, pregnancy, childbirth, and female physiology at the time.

In book 7, chapter 16, Bernard goes on to describe a natural birth (head first after seven to eleven or more months [*sic*] of pregnancy) and what constitutes an unnatural birth: any presentation other than head first. He then lists the reasons for a protracted birth and the symptoms by which one can recognize whether the feuts is dead. The reasons for difficult labor are divided into intrinsic and extrinsic. Bernard thus follows tradition. Among the extrinsic are excessive heat or cold, an inept midwife, a premature birth, an existing scar, or constipation.[110] Intrinsic reasons are a prepubescent conception and the consequent narrow birth canal; obesity; extreme fear and delicacy on the part of the mother; a too large, too delicate, or dead fetus; two heads, or twins; unnatural presentation; or a small or too dry uterus. If none of the above applies, the reason has to be sought in the secundines (placenta).

The signs by which a dead fetus is signaled are facial discoloration and fetid breath; pain and immobility in the abdomen, Bernard specifies, are good reasons for increased vigilance. Bernard's remarks about the midwife's tasks and qualities recall some details of Soranus's *Gynecology,* notably the long and slim fingers required of a midwife. She is the one to deal with difficult labor through baths and fomentations, unguents and manual dilation of the cervix. In the case of an obstructing scar, surgical instruments should be used to open it.[111]

In Bernard's *Lilium,* then, the textual environment of the operation is that of obstetrics, but in practice the operation belonged to surgery. In the work of Guy de Chauliac we find somewhat more explicit instructions regarding the performance of a Caesarean section. Guy was one of the greatest surgeons of his century; he was trained at Montpellier and Bologna, traveled widely in his profession, and finally, about 1348, at the time of the great plague, became surgeon to Pope Clement VI in Avignon. In 1359 he was named provost of the chapter of Saint-Just in Lyons. He was highly regarded by several popes and at the time of his death in 1368 had just been honored once more by Pope Urban V.

Guy deals with the postmortem Caesarean in chapter 7 of the sixth treatise of his *Grande chirurgie.* He first lists possible reasons for a difficult birth: wrong presentation of the fetus (the only natural one is head first) and multiple births (Avicenna mentions quintuplets, Guy informs his readers; Abulcasis, even ten children born at one time); but, he adds, since it is mostly women who occupy themselves with such things it is hardly worth spending too much time on these questions. However, one should tell midwives (*obstetrices*) that if the birth is difficult despite normal presentation, unguents should be used to soften the birth canal. The woman herself should help by pressing, by holding her breath, and by sneezing, which might be induced by pepper or other substances. Cyclamen tied to the thigh facilitates the birth (say the experts). To correct unnatural presentation Guy recommends version of the unborn through external manipulation, for example, raising the thighs of the woman. He does not mention internal version, as did Soranus and others, possibly because his confidence in the midwives' abilities is limited. Should the child die before delivery the midwife must try to extract the child either by hand (anointed with unguents) or by induced sneezing. Medicines with abortive powers (for example, castor, myrrh, and others) are recommended. If nothing works, the child should be extracted by hooks "entier ou en pièces."

Should it happen that the woman dies and the child is still alive—and as the king's order forbids burial of a pregnant woman before the child is extracted—one should hold open the mouth and the uterus of the woman (as the women—that is, midwives and female attendants—desire it) and make an incision with a razor along the left side, since this side is freer than the right side because of the liver. Through insertion of the fingers the child can then be pulled out.[112]

These instructions, of a purely practical nature, combine much of what we saw in such texts as Soranus's *Gynecology*. Guy also revives some forgotten techniques. The extraction by mutilating hooks, for example, had not been mentioned in detail since the period of Arabic obstetrics.[113] But he also displays anatomical knowledge (position of the liver), some legal wisdom, and familiarity with learned legends. Even though this obstetrical chapter constitutes only a minute part of Guy's gigantic work and even though he denigrates female practitioners, some real concern seems to come through in the passages just summarized. For the first time a surgical instrument is specified; for the first time instructions as to the position of the incision are given.[114] These innovations may reflect a concern for the improvement of the operating techniques of lay persons, notably midwives. They may also mark a step on the way to the medicalization of obstetrics and reflect the growing interest of male surgeons in this exclusively female domain.

It is only a few decades later that we encounter the first surgeon who in his writings lays claim to having performed a Caesarean and an embryotomy (after a Caesarean?) himself. Piero d'Argellata (d. 1423), a professor at Bologna and the author of *Chirurgia*, writes about the extraction of the fetus in chapter 7 of book 5, treatise 19. He follows Guy de Chauliac in many of his obstetrical remarks and also recommends the postmortem Caesarean: "One should hold open the mother's mouth as well as the uterus so that air can enter and the child can come out. The woman should be opened with a razor along the left side of the abdomen. . . . Some time ago I prudently made the incision along the *linea alba* up to the breast bone. Neither the intestine nor the child was touched and in this way I extracted the child".[115] It is also possible to extract a dead child in this manner: the "perforation" is then held open by hooking the fingers along the incision, and the child is pulled out. Piero says, "*Ego aliquando feci*" (*I once made*) and "*extraxi*" (*I extracted*), clearly indicating that he performed the operation himself and did not relegate it to a midwife.

This innovative male presence is a fifteenth-century phenomenon. Giovanni Michele Savonarola (d. 1466), who wrote a gynecological treatise in Italian, also recommends expert medical (that is, male) help when the future mother is a *domina magna,* or a wealthy woman. He limits these male consultations ("for poor people the doctor does not labor much"),[116] but his recommendation nevertheless lets us discern the trend toward male participation in obstetrical procedures—a trend that was undoubtedly arrested by one obstacle, concisely expressed by Savonarola: generally, obstetrics was not one of the more lucrative branches of medicine.

Alessandro Benedetti (1450–1525) also recommended a postmortem Caesarean in chapter 15 ("De obstetricis officio") of his *De re medica.* Benedetti was a surgeon and anatomist from Bologna who, despite his reliance on the ancient authorities, managed to make some new discoveries, such as the vaginal glands later named after Bertholin.[117] That it is again a surgeon who mentions the Caesarean is worthy of note.

In Germany, the situation was somewhat different. Midwifery there was subjected to official control in the form of statutes, usually issued by city councils, about a century earlier than in France (mid-fifteenth century versus about 1560). One of these statutes, dating from about 1480, comes from southern Germany and describes in great detail how a Caesarean should be performed. This text is unusually explicit:

> Many mothers ask, when they feel that they are dying, to liberate the child by an incision. In that case, the skillful midwife has to open up one side, but not the right one; for in men the heart is located on the left side, but in women on the right side. She shall start cutting in the lower part of the belly around the pubic bone, about the width of one hand. With her oiled hand she must carefully move aside the entrails. The sick woman shall lie on her back with her head tilted back so that she can reach the uterus. After the opening of the uterus the woman should be tilted to one side, as the midwives know well. The child should be freed from the fetal membranes. But the woman, if she still seems to be alive, should be turned again on her back. The wound should be closed with three or four ligatures by means of a needle and a silk or other thread. On top of this should be placed a plaster

made from three eggs and some fabric of strong hemp to which one may add, when available, some Armenian clay (*bolus armenicus*). The plaster should be tied onto the wound. The woman receives a sip of the best wine. Should she survive and regain consciousness, give her a drink made of the roots of salsify and of mountain albanum sautéed in wine. And the woman will recover with God's help.[118]

These instructions are clearly addressed to midwives and seem to assume a fair chance of the woman's survival. In reality, however, this chance was minimal, given the danger of infection.

One of the most important German texts of this period, Eucharius Roesslin's 1513 *Der Swangern Frawen vnd Hebammen Rosegarten* (The pregnant women's and midwives' rose garden), is essentially a compilation of ancient texts on obstetrics. It starts right off with remarks on fetal positions and practical advice to midwives. Nevertheless, the identity of its addressees is ambiguous; they could be either male readers or female midwives. Still, the passage on Caesarean birth at the end of chapter 9 seems to be meant specifically for his (presumably male) reader. For whereas other instructions are prefaced by "the midwife should," in the passage on Caesareans Roesslin says, "*You* should" (soltu = sollst *du*).[119] In any case, Roesslin's passages on the Caesarean section are an exact translation of Guy de Chauliac: he specifies the position of the incision (on the left, since on the right side is the liver); the instrument: a *Schermesser* (razor); the necessity to hold open the mother's mouth (also the uterus and the vagina [in an addition to Chauliac]); the removal of the child by hand; the reference to Julius Caesar's birth. Compared with the midwifery text just cited the instructions here are very scanty and of limited practical value. And yet, Roesslin makes an effort to get away from the even more useless type of natural history exemplified by the pseudo-Albertus Magnus's *Secreta mulierum,* which repeated ancient lore on astrology, conception, embryology, obstetrics, and the nature of women and thus was really an encyclopedia of what passed then as natural philosophy rather than of medicine.

One of the characteristics of texts preceding Roesslin was that they did not treat obstetrics as a separate discipline. It was seen either as part of surgery or in the wider framework of female physiology. Because Roesslin addressed himself in the vernacular specifically to midwives (through the probable intermediary of a literate male surgeon), he has always been hailed as *the* teacher of midwives in Europe. His attitude toward midwives was on the whole more positive and trusting than that of Guy de

Chauliac, as can be seen through a minute change in the German text. Where Guy treats the holding open of the mouth (in reality a useless procedure) as a concession to the attending women, Roesslin sees the midwives' experience in a positive light when he says: "as women usually know well" (*als die frawen gewonlich wol wissen*). The German version of the *Secreta mulierum,* which antedates Roesslin by about sixty years, had contributed to the perpetuation of this idea in its short passage on Casearean section: "the mother's mouth should be held open with a little piece of wood and the fruit should be cut out of her body."[120] In any case, Roesslin tries to put some value on traditional beliefs of midwifery.

Despite some observations on present-day practices (notably on the birth stools common in Germany and France, in chapter 4) Roesslin's *Rosegarten,* like most medieval medical treatises, was steeped in preceding textual traditions rather than first-hand experience. But things began to change with the next generation of surgeon-authors, especially in France.

FRANÇOIS ROUSSET AND THE CONTROVERSY OVER CAESAREANS ON LIVING WOMEN

The group around Ambroise Paré, one of the greatest surgeons of the sixteenth century, was responsible for a new approach—and a new rhetoric—in obstetrical writings. Most of his writings rely heavily on the ancients, but occasionally personal experience surfaces, if not always explicitly.

Paré's theoretical objections to Caesareans on living women seem to have been based on the unfortunate experiences of his pupil and colleague Jacques Guillemeau, who performed several fatal Caesareans under his supervision.[121] In his writings Paré does not mention any personal experience when he discusses postmortem Caesarean section.[122] He especially insists on the speed with which such an operation has to be performed, since the child will have no way to breathe after the mother's death. He rejects the ideas that opening the mother's mouth and vagina could enable the child to breathe.[123] The most important paragraph of this chapter is the last, in which he gives his reasons for rejecting Caesareans on living women:

> I am surprised that there are people who claim to have seen women who, in order to be delivered of their children, had their abdomens cut open, not

only once but several times. This seems impossible to me, since, in order to extract the child, a large incision has to be made in the muscles of the epigastrum and also in the uterus, which is so imbued with blood that a fatal hemorrhage would be the result. In addition, once the wound closes the scar would prevent the uterus from ever dilating again. . . . I will never advise this procedure, which involves such great danger and offers no hope.[124]

It was this type of objection that Rousset addressed in the preface to his famous treatise, *Traitté nouveau de l'hystérotomotokie, ou enfantement Caesarien* (1581). As a consequence of Rousset's work a bitter controversy erupted about the advisability of Caesareans on living women.[125] In the 1590s Rousset became the target of vitriolic attacks by Jacques Marchant and of somewhat more temperate attacks by Guillemeau. What was it in Rousset's treatise that aroused such strong passions and strong language?

The subtitle of Rousset's work indicates the revolutionary nature of his remarks: *Extraction de l'enfant par incision latérale du ventre, et matrice de la femme grosse ne pouvant autrement accoucher. Et ce sans preiudicier à la vie de l'un, ny de l'autre; ny empescher la foecondité maternelle par après* (The extraction of the child through a lateral incision of the abdomen and uterus of a pregnant woman who cannot otherwise give birth. And that without endangering the life of the one or the other and without preventing subsequent maternal fertility). The claim made in the last part of this subtitle went against all accepted medical wisdom of the time. Rousset is aware of this—and especially Paré's objections—when, in the part "Au Lecteur," he makes a reference to some "amiable disputes" he had with Paré over the birth, which he (Rousset) baptized "enfantement Caesarien." Nevertheless, in the first edition of Rousset's work Paré's approving signature can be found right next to that of the dean of the Faculty of Medicine, a testimony to an at least ambiguous attitude on Paré's part toward the feasibility of a successful Caesarean.[126] About a century later, François Mauriceau explained Paré's ambiguity on that subject by saying that this was "because he will not have posterity know that he was able to consent to so great a cruelty."[127]

Some of the ideological underpinnings of Rousset's thought are evident in the "Sonnet de l'autheur au lecteur chirurgien" (Sonnet of the author for the reader-surgeon) at the beginning of the treatise. Here he equates a difficult birth with the Gordian knot. Just as Alexander undid the knot with his sword ("au Couteau"), so the courageous surgeon should undo the "knot" of childbirth with his knife. The reward will not be all of Asia, as it was for Alexander, but the happiness of having given life to mothers and children ("et eux de toy tiendront la vie"). How radical and heroic the operation was for Rousset could not be better expressed than in the image of Alexander cutting through the Gordian knot. I believe that Rousset's texts can be read as a cry of protest against the general impression that male participation in obstetrics always involved death. Or, as Wilson puts it, "the task of the midwife was to deliver a *living* child, the task of the male practitioner a *dead* one."[128]

Rousset was aware of the novelty of his ideas. "Something unheard of, never written about, hardly credible to those who see it" is how he describes his subject in the prefatory epistle. Here he also justifies his using French instead of Latin by dedicating it to the poor women who must otherwise die without help and to surgeons whose Latin may not be excellent. He explains that a more ample treatise in Latin is to follow.[129] Remarkably, the Latin translation by Caspar Bauhin was much more successful and saw many more editions than Rousset's French text. His intended audience clearly did not buy his treatise; he found his real audience among the learned physicians and those surgeons whose Latin was "excellent."

The text begins with a definition of a Caesarean (extraction of a child—either alive or dead—through the side of the mother by incision of the epigastrum and the uterus) and a refusal to speak of postmortem Caesareans (known already to the ancients). Rousset also explains the name of the operation by a reference to the "first of the Caesars who was Scipio Africanus," supposedly born this way. Thus Rousset does not subscribe to the legend of Julius Caesar's birth by Caesarean but, by creating the medical term, nevertheless kept this erroneous idea alive, since most people are aware only of the term and not of Rousset's explanation.

Rousset then lists the indications for a Caesarean section: if the child is too large or malformed or dead (in that case it may too bloated to be extracted by natural means); in the case of twins or of problematic presentation. Other indications concern the mother: if, through reasons of extreme youth or old age, she is too narrow or "hard," that is, not elastic enough.[130]

In the next section Rousset takes on the age-old tension between theory and practice as well as between the representatives of school medicine and those of rural practice. Since none of the ancients has written on the subject of Caesareans, learned doctors and surgeons give no credit to the practice, although operations of this kind have been and are being performed by rural barbers, if very rarely. Therefore—and here Rousset defines his rhetorical method—three means will be used to persuade the skeptics: experience (through case histories); pertinent reasons (through discussion of medical points); sufficient authority (discussion of possible analogies, wounds of a character similar to a Caesarean incision that have indeed been dealt with by the ancient authorities).[131]

As a preface to his case histories, Rousset describes his method of gathering evidence. He basically relies on the testimonies of "gens fidèles" (trustworthy people) and of "personnages non suspects."[132] In other words, Rousset never performed the operation himself and was not even present at most of the cases he describes.

The first case concerns a woman named Anne Godart who gave birth by Caesarean six times in a row. At the seventh birth she died because her surgeon, Nicolas Guillet, had died some time before and no other surgeon was willing to perform the operation. In the second case, Rousset wanted to go and see the woman, who had delivered three times by Caesarean, but she died of the plague before he could get his first-hand testimony. The next two cases all concern multiple successful Caesareans, news of which was transmitted to Rousset by letter. Now a break occurs in the narrative. The next section is headed "Histoires oculaires" (Eyewitness stories). Rousset addresses the "ami lecteur" and defends himself against accusations of being inept, boring, and too concerned with particulars. The only way to get to the truth of matters, he says, lies in just such particulars. The next two stories involve Rousset directly. In the first, he examined a woman with a ventral hernia who explained that the long scar on her left side was the trace of a successful Caesarean performed seven years earlier by an old barber of her village. Rousset had intended to contact this barber but was, "through the difficulty of the times," unable to find the piece of paper on which he had written his name. Rousset's wish to "gather from him practical details gained from experience" remained unfulfilled. In the next case, Rousset actually witnessed the performance of the operation that he himself had advised for a woman in prolonged labor. Since the experienced surgeon Ambroise le Noir could not be found, a young barber ("le premier trouvé") performed the operation. Here we learn the exact date (Easter 1556) and the way the incision was made: on the right side about one finger down from the navel. The barber was so skillful that little blood was shed, and he managed to pull out the living child and the afterbirth. He then closed the wound with five stitches (he did not suture the uterus) and after forty days' bed rest the woman was well again. She later gave birth to a daughter naturally.[133]

The next cases concern the excision of dead fetuses. Here Rousset accuses several midwives who through their incompetence "broke up" a poor woman in such a way that, despite the successful removal of the fetus, she was ill for seven months. Similar remarks appear in the story of one Jeanne Michel, who was tormented by midwives without any result until, in the tenth month of pregnancy, she was finally delivered of a dead fetus.[134]

One thought is paramount in Rousset's writings: he wants to overcome the resistance to the operation on the part of medical practitioners. He encourages surgeons, such as Adam Aubry, not to waste time through cowardly reflections but to go ahead with a Caesarean as quickly as possible.[135]

Of the 228 pages of Rousset's treatise only 17 are devoted to case histories of successful Caesareans. One of the most dramatic stories of a successful Caesarean is not in Rousset's work proper but in the appendix to Bauhin's Latin translation of Rousset. It is that of Jacob Nufer, a Swiss pig gelder who, in the year 1500, delivered his wife surgically after she had been in labor for several days. Great drama accompanied this operation, for Nufer first had to get the permission of the authorities, and courageous midwives had to be found (only two out of the thirteen he approached finally decided to assist this determined man). With a single deep cut he opened the uterus ("as if operating on a pig") and extracted the child at the first try. He then sewed up his wife in the same manner he used for his animals, and it was only then that the eleven timid midwives were allowed back into the room. The following year his wife supposedly gave birth to twins (without a Caesarean). Should this story be true it would indeed be remarkable. It is unlikely that Nufer sutured the uterus. In fact, Rousset specifies in several stories that surgeons did not suture the uterus.[136] Some historians have doubted that Nufer performed a Caesarean at all and assert that his wife's pregnancy must have been extra-uterine. Two factors argue against this, however, according to Pietro Gall: the mother's extended labor and the good health of the child.[137] In the absence of asepsis and anaesthetics in this period the mother's survival in this as in all of Rousset's stories must be seen as a fortunate accident.

The second and third parts of Rousset's treatise contain an operating manual (where, for example, he compares a Caesarean with the operation to remove bladder stones), while the fourth part speaks of the dangerous alternatives to a Caesarean in complications such as a retained and putrid fetus, abcesses of the uterus or the hypogastrium (through extrauterine pregnancies). His point here is that in every case an extraction by incision poses the smallest risk. Here again, Rousset uses numerous case histories, some of them in letters addressed to him, to buttress his arguments. He defends himself repeatedly against allegations that his cases took place far away; to counter certain attacks he tells some stories that happened closer to Paris, as if this geographical proximity guaranteed the stories' veracity.[138] Part 5 deals with experimental surgery (specifically the removal of the uterus in animals without any adverse effect), and part 6 explains that a Caesarean does not impede a woman's fertility.

Rousset's treatise is remarkable for its passionate tone and polemical stance. Acerbic remarks on the incompetency of midwives stand side by side with accusations against the cowardly passivity of many surgeons. Radical innovation and active intervention in childbirth are his tenets, which did not endear him to the established medical community. According to Young, Rousset's work "was a masterpiece, and he appears to be the first writer who had the courage to advise the performance of the operation upon a living woman." Pundel also lauds Rousset for his theoretical descriptions (many of which are still true today), although he doubts that under sixteenth-century conditions Rousset's recommendations could have ensured the success of the operation.[139]

But apparently it was exactly the courage praised by Young that made Rousset the target of a series of more and more vicious attacks by his colleagues, especially Jacques Marchant.[140] Jacques Marchant's first *Declamatio* (2) was directed against Rousset's *Dialogus* of 1590 (1), in which the latter refuted all the accusations that had been leveled against his treatise of 1581. Written as an imaginary dialogue between two characters named Sozometer and Catagelastes, the *Dialogus* begins with an opposition of darkness and light, the light representing, of course, more enlightened medical views. Sozometer insists on the novelty of what he (Rousset) had written about Caesarean section and supports his remarks by some more case histories. These examples, he says, have been unjustly attacked. Interesting in the context of the question of possible audiences for medical treatises is the defense of writing in French: "Gallus ego, ad Gallos, de Gallis, Gallica scripsi" (I am French, I have written for Frenchmen, about Frenchmen, in French), says Sozometer. And why should he not write in French, since all the ancients wrote in their own languages? In addition, as usefulness is one of the aims of a medical treatise, the French language lends itself better to this aim. (The *Dialogus* itself, of course, being a polemical tract and not a practical handbook, is in Latin.) Sozometer admits that the ancients did not speak of Caesarean section, but in general terms, he adds, they advocated that "what could be done, should be done." His counterattack against famous and mendacious doctors who condemned his innovations and his use of case histories culminates in the enumeration of the empty trappings these professionals care for, namely "tituli, gemmae, toga, pilea, otia privatae, nomine dicta gradus" (titles, jewels, clothes, hats, leisure time, and to be addressed by their degrees). Caesareans are not popular with this kind of doctor because a successful operation brings very little praise and its failure great blame.[141] The *Dialogus* ends with an attempt to counter Paré's accusations of Rousset's being an impostor who should revoke his writings. In a long series of classical examples one point is illustrated again and again: that one has to show initiative and courage for innovative procedures even at the risk of being maligned and misunderstood.

Clearly, the *Dialogus* failed to convince Jacques Marchant. Marchant first refutes Rousset's observations on the analogy between the Caesarean operation and procedures that can safely be done on animals (the fifth part of Rousset's treatise) and then goes on to use the same arguments as Paré to demonstrate the impossibility of a successful Caesarean: the large wound in the epigastric muscles, the loss of blood from the uterus and its fatal consequences. Therefore, he says, this dangerous and desperate procedure should never be undertaken. After a whole list of examples of unsuccessful Caesareans recounted by various witnesses, Marchant addresses himself directly to Rousset: "Cannot the above examples bring you to revoke your *sententia*? No," he answers for himself, "you are too obstinate."[142]

Marchant also raises the fundamental question of "natural" versus "unnatural" childbirth by appealing to the concepts of nature, tradition, and practice. How can a surgeon show so much temerity, he asks, to plunge his hands into the side of a pregnant woman, when nature indicates a natural way of exit? In addition, of the learned ancients not one mentioned Casearean section in his writings. As for practice, Marchant points out that women are very patient in childbirth and that therefore it would be better to wait for a natural birth rather than to rush into a desperate and doomed operation. Against male involvement in obstetrics he puts forward that women are so much more experienced in the "mysteries of Lucina."[143]

The rhetoric of this part of Marchant's texts is still rather moderate. So is that of Guillemeau's letter to Rousset inserted in the first *Declamatio*. "We are not categorically against innovations," he claims, "but only against those that are horrible. But as to your small and inept collection of writings—I shall be silent on that topic." Guillemeau seems to have checked up on some of Rousset's eyewitnesses and have found them to be lying. To dramatize his points Guillemeau draws on his own experience of several failures in attempting Caesareans on living women, "done according to your specifications under monsieur Paré." The moving descriptions of the women's deaths culminate in an ardent plea against the operation as envisaged by Rousset.[144]

It is in *Declamatio III* that Marchant's attack against Rousset becomes vicious. "Absurda, nugatoria, incredibilis" are the adjectives he uses to describe Rousset's so-called eyewitness stories. "How easy it is to hallucinate," he exclaims, "and thus to become the source of all errors. And this is what you have become, the creator of this plague which is sweeping Europe. You are nothing but a fraud." "Your beloved Caesar [that is, Caesarean section] now lies extinct in Europe," Marchant claims, undoubtedly alluding to the success his (Marchant's) writings had in dissuading surgeons from the operation. "And," he adds triumphantly, "to name this operation Caesarean section, was a disservice to your hero. You should have named it after the cruel Tarquinius who delighted in the blood and death of women." And Marchant goes on to write an imaginary inscription for Caesar's tomb that begins, "What lies here? Caesarean birth." There follows the death sentence for the operation, which is called "puer infoelix" (unfortunate boy).[145]

In *Carmen,* the poem that follows *Declamatio III,* Marchant reiterates his condemnation: "Caesarean birth is not reasonable and certainly not a remedy but rather a dangerous procedure which belongs to the 'ars carnificum.'"[146] Against such an accumulation of passionate attacks Rousset could, in his final *Responsio* (7), do little more than repeat what he had said previously in his original treatise and the *Dialogus.*

During this heated exchange of views on the feasibility of Caesarean sections on living women an Italian doctor named Scipione Mercurio returned from a long trip to France and started to describe his experiences in his *Commare o raccoglitrice.*[147] As early as 1571 and 1572 learned doctors told him that in cases where the fetus was too large one could help pregnant women by an incision that could be made either in the right or the left side. No danger existed for the mother or child. "This," Mercurio admits, "did not seem impossible to me." Having never seen such an operation, Mercurio sought out a surgeon near Toulouse who went with him to see two women who had had Caesareans. One of them told

Mercurio that she became pregnant again after the Caesarean and that this birth presented no problems. But, as for most of Rousset's cases, Mercurio saw the scars only after the fact. Nevertheless, he became an advocate of Caesareans on living women (but only if they were strong), especially after reading Rousset. Like Rousset, he asserts that "this remedy (the Caesarean operation) does not belong in the realm of midwifery but into that of the doctor or learned surgeon," but only if he is "experienced, courageous, prudent and, above all, has a thorough knowledge of anatomy."[148]

Mercurio developed his own theories concerning the Caesarean birth and, like Rousset, he used the analogy of operations for bladder stones to demonstrate its feasibility. Today Mercurio is probably best known as the first medical writer to name a narrow pelvis as an indication for a Caesarean and as the only surgeon who took Rousset's side in his own writings.

From a modern perspective, both sides in the quarrel about Caesareans on living women were right and wrong. In Young's judgment, Rousset's treatise was a masterpiece; Newell, as well, while claiming that most of the pregnancies observed by Rousset must have been extrauterine, concedes that "this treatise had one great merit in that it brought the operation to the attention of the medical profession and suggested the possibility of its performance on living women."[149] But, of course, given the conditions prevailing in the practice of medicine at Rousset's time, his advice was close to foolhardy, and Marchant's passionate rejection of Rousset seems justified. Nevertheless, Rousset made a case for medical innovation and initiative that was to bear its fruits many centuries later.

In this chapter I have placed the Caesarean section in the context of pregnancy and birth in the medieval period as well as in the context of medical writings on these subjects. Outside of the medical literature and some religious writings, little attention was given to these profoundly female functions. Birth was a little-valued and dangerous process in which the Caesarean operation represented the extreme, that is fatal, outcome.

The most important factor for the emergence of Caesarean birth as a medical procedure was the laicization of surgery, which prompted a new consciousness of professional competency on the part of the medical and surgical professions. The performance of dissections made possible new views about opening up the human body. The close alliance of theory and practice in Montpellier, and especially Bernard of Gordon's interest in matters conveyed to him by "old wives" and in *artificia* (more practice-oriented than that of his predecessors), led him to include the operation in his *Lilium*. Before the fourteenth century, Caesarean birth had been recommended purely in a religious context: midwives were urged to perform the operation in order to baptize the newborn.

The controversy about whether to perform a Caesarean on a living woman illustrated a surge of medical optimism—albeit limited to a few individuals, especially François Rousset—in the late sixteenth century that was quickly checked a few decades later. From a theoretical and ideological perspective, Rousset and Marchant provided us with discussions on concepts of nature, tradition, and practice that illuminate important currents in Renaissance medicine.

Most important, male surgeons, motivated by scientific, professional, and probably also by financial interests, began to perform Caesarean sections around 1400. Thus it was through Caesarean birth that they entered the field of obstetrics, and they did so much earlier than previously thought.

The close connection between birth and death that existed in the Middle Ages is most dramatically highlighted in Caesarean birth; let us now turn to the images that show us women—both mothers and midwives—confronted by the ultimate threat in which two lives hang in the balance: death in childbirth.

2 CAESAREAN BIRTH IN THE ARTISTIC IMAGINATION

What can pictures tell us about medieval life and society and about the attitudes and feelings of medieval men and women? What is their meaning and how is their meaning related to the conditions of their production? What kind of relationship do pictures have to the texts they illustrate? How do they reflect the tension between iconographic tradition and realistic observation? Many of these questions have been the subject of scholarly debate in recent years and are especially important in the context of medical iconography.[1]

Illustrations of childbirth come from both medical and nonmedical manuscripts and thus represent a variety of approaches to the depiction of domestic and medical scenes. Pictures of Caesarean birth, many of them showing the birth of Julius Caesar, constitute a new and fecund source for the study of medieval iconographic development as well as for the recovery of women's history. Although a few of these images have been reproduced before (mostly in summary histories of Caesarean section), their importance for the history of gender roles in the medical profession has not been recognized.

To observe medieval women at work is not an easy task. The documentation is fragmentary, and whole areas of women's activities, such as domestic and farm labor, left few traces in medieval—and for that matter modern—historiography.[2] Women doctors and midwives left more traces than peasant women did, but it is difficult to evaluate the records that survived. A large number of these records are negative in the sense that many women healers appeared in records only when they were brought to trial on charges of illegal practice or witchcraft; others, especially the very few female physicians, are little more than names in various registers. The situation is hardly better for midwives. Before the fourteenth century, few texts dealt with their tasks, and when midwives and their activities finally appear more frequently in historical documents it is in the context of the witch-hunts. In order to sort out the blurry and often conflicting images of medieval midwives, I will first analyze the pictorial evidence and then—in the next chapter—turn to the texts. Comparing and contrasting these two different types of sources should bring us a step closer to understanding how women functioned in one of the most important professions open to them in the Middle Ages: midwifery.[3] The area of Caesarean birth crystallized many of the problems confronting medieval midwives. The representations of midwives and male surgeons at work at Caesarean sections reflect and evaluate their professional competence in a critical situation as well as their compassion toward mother and child.[4]

An important feature of the iconographic evidence for Caesarean births is that it exists in a *series* of images ranging from the late thirteenth to the sixteenth century. Such a rich series of illustrations showing the same medical procedure is extremely rare in medical iconography. Obviously, it is much more valuable to trace the evolution of a given medical scene than to use one image as an illustration regardless of the specific work or period it comes from, as has been done in previous studies of Caesarean section. Second, images of Caesarean birth appear in nonmedical texts and are thus situated at the crossroads of two iconographic traditions that I will consider in turn: birth scenes in medical and in nonmedical manuscripts. For each tradition, I will discuss the relationship of the pictures both to the texts they illustrate and to what we can know of the medical practice and the social reality of the time. One important focus of this discussion is of course the depiction of women— both as patients and healers—and of their relationship to male participants in the birth scenes.[5]

QUESTIONS OF PRODUCTION AND INTERPRETATION

A case has been made recently for the division of sources into women's, men's, and common sources, especially with regard to medieval sources on childbirth.[6] What type of source is the iconography of Caesarean birth? Who conceived these images of suffering or dead mothers and their female or male attendants? Although we cannot hope for certainty in answering these questions we can nevertheless engage in some informed speculation as to the circumstances in which pictures of Caesarean births were produced.

Women participated in medieval book production and trade in a variety of ways. Most of the evidence for medieval women acting as painters or illuminators is iconographic and comes principally from manuscripts of Boccaccio's *De claris mulieribus* and the reworking of it by Christine de Pizan in the *Livre de la cité des dames*. As Christine's book is written in praise of women's capabilities to do just about anything, it is hardly surprising to see them pursue all kinds of professions in the illuminations. Whether they were able to practice these professions in real life is a different question.

In the late thirteenth century a woman, Perronnelle d'Auteuil, appeared in the Paris tax rolls in connection with a workshop for books. Her title was *imagière*, a term that could refer "to a painter, sculptor, or even an architect."[7] Perronnelle was a widow and probably took over her husband's workshop, which she managed to run at a profit. In this way medieval women often were able to enter professions ordinarily closed to them. Some even worked on the side as *libraires*, that is "one who acted as an agent for selling books left on deposit but who also might rent out master copies from which other copies might be made."[8] The daughter of the famous illuminator Jean le Noir worked together with her father in fourteenth-century Flanders and Paris. Christine de Pizan praised a contemporary illuminator named Anastasia. It is impossible to say, however, which parts of the illuminator's work these women performed. Different specialists probably worked together on the more elaborate miniatures.[9] Anastasia, for example, was especially known for her skill in painting manuscript borders and miniature backgrounds, which suggests that women may have specialized in these techniques but did not often tackle full-fledged miniatures. In any case, women were present in and sometimes even owned workshops that illuminated books. How much they had to do with the conceptualization of a given manuscript cannot be determined. For the manuscripts discussed in this chapter, some of the artists' names are known and all were men.[10]

It must be assumed, therefore, that most of the illustrations considered here were painted by men. Since ordinary men were in general not admitted at births, the illuminators must have received their information regarding Caesarean birth scenes from someone else, probably from midwives and, for the later centuries, from surgeons. It is unlikely that female illuminators could have given their male colleagues the medical details regarding the procedure—that is, the instruments used for a Caesarean and the location of the incision—that are reflected in the pictures. They could have filled them in on the atmosphere in the birth chamber and the circumstances of a normal birth, but probably a Caesarean was seldom witnessed by women not in a healing or serving profession.

It is certain that there must have been some female-male collaboration, and this collaboration could have created what Jacobsen would call a common source, a feature that greatly increases our chance of getting a more objective picture of the respective activities of female midwives and male surgeons.

One of the problems in interpreting ancient images is that their meaning is seldom univocal. For early Christian frescoes, for example, Margaret Miles has shown recently that the language of images does not allow for one "detachable conclusion."[11] The images of the fourth-century Roman churches she discusses can be read either as inviting pagans to join the Christian faith or as a representation of the exclusiveness of the early church. The function of women in fourteenth-century Tuscan painting is similarly multivocal. Miles suggests that the idealized passive attitudes of women in many of these paintings contrasted quite sharply with the roles Italian women came to play in the urban society of the fourteenth century. The depiction of women as helpless diaphanous beings thus may have enabled men to ignore or suppress the increasing importance of women. But Miles also warns against forcing our modern points of view on medieval pictures. The idealization of a woman's virginal qualities, for instance, does not necessarily speak only of sexual repression. A spiritualization of the body may have given some comfort to medieval women who had to face the reality of sexual dependency and frequent childbearing.[12] Similarly, Penny Schine Gold has found that changing representations of the relationship between Christ and the Virgin Mary do not reflect a shift in attitudes toward real medieval women but rather signal a variety of interpretive possibilities characterized by ambiguity and even contradictions.[13]

These observations are meant to serve as a caveat against any ideologically biased interpretation of medieval images depicting women. In order to present a clear view of the significance of the series of Caesarean birth scenes, I will trace the traditions of medical iconography and the place of medical and nonmedical illustrations of childbirth within these traditions.

TRADITIONS IN MEDICAL ILLUSTRATION

The earliest examples of medical illustrations probably date back to the fourth or third century B.C. They were not illustrations of medical practice but probably schematic figures used by Alexandrian anatomists. From the Hellenistic period dates the famous five-picture cycle, in which every element shows one organic system: muscles, nerves, organs, arteries and veins. A sixth picture showing a pregnant woman may also have belonged to this cycle.[14] The five- (or six-) picture cycle made its way via Byzantium and Persia to medieval Europe. It forms part of a group of schematic illustrations that can be found in countless medical manuscripts. One of these schemata is the zodiac man (or woman) who has a zodiac sign assigned to every part of his or her body, indicating the dependency of a particular organ on one of the signs. Guided by this system, a physician would decide on the propitious and unpropitious periods for treating or operating on a given organ.[15] This connection of astrology and medicine was one of the important characteristics of medieval medicine.

Other schematic human figures show the bloodletting man and the cautery man. Phlebotomy and cauterization were by far the most widespread forms of medical intervention in the Middle Ages. Medieval practitioners thus needed practical advice on where to make incisions for bloodletting and on the location of the points for cauterization. These two figures, as well as the spectacular wound man—transpierced by swords and arrows—belong to the practice-oriented area of medical illustrations.[16] So do most of the illustrations in surgical treatises, such as the famous fourteenth-century manuscript of Roger Frugardi's *Chirurgia* in the British Library (Sloane 1977). This often-reproduced manuscript shows a variety of surgical procedures in an interesting iconographic arrangement: the upper band of illuminations depicts the life of Christ, the lower compartments feature the surgeon at work.[17]

A physician's (not very successful) activities are chronicled in an extraordinary series of illuminations inserted in a late-thirteenth-century manuscript at the Bodleian Library in Oxford.[18] This case history follows an unfortunate lady from her first fainting spell to her death. As her doctor tries to give her some medication, the lady's companions and (clerical?) attendants seem to counsel against his prescriptions. The rejection of treatment results in a relapse, and the urinalysis in picture number 5 spells disaster: the physician drops the vial in a hopeless gesture. The lady dies and the physician has nothing left to do but to preside over the autopsy of his patient, which is performed by a knife-wielding man in a short robe that identifies him as a "low surgeon." This illustration may well be the earliest surviving image of an anatomical dissection.[19] The whole cycle possibly has a moralizing intent:[20] it exhorts patients to follow their physicians' advice rather than that of their foolish companions and attendants.

This lively pictorial narrative leads us to the obvious question of how realistic medical illustrations were. Which influence was stronger: iconographic models or realistic observation? The strength of iconographic tradition as well as the interdependence of medical and nonmedical illustrations are discussed in Heide Grape-Albers's important work *Spätantike Bilder aus der Welt des Arztes,* on late antique medical illustration and its transmission to the Middle Ages. She makes a strong case for the iconographic dependence of most medieval medical illustrations on antique and late antique sources. A striking example of the analogies that can be found between the profane iconography of late antiquity and early Christian art is the schema of a physician standing next to a patient's bed. The same pattern serves to illustrate Aeneas's dream in a late antique Virgil manuscript as well as several healing scenes showing Jesus as a physician in fourteenth-century manuscripts of the Bible.[21]

Karl Sudhoff, one of the greatest historians of medieval medicine, takes a different position.[22] According to him, only the earlier surgical illustrations of the Middle Ages still show a strong dependency on antique (Hellenistic) models, which they often reproduce unchanged. Starting with the thirteenth century, however, new elements are introduced that are culled from observation rather than exclusively from an iconographic tradition. This type of illustration starts to replace the traditional images, and whole series of illustrations are created from scratch. The illustrators employ the dominant formal elements of their time, but in general the medical illustrator is less dependent on traditional schemata than the illuminator of hagiographic legends or historical texts. In the latter, there is a much stronger constraint with regard to the iconographic tradition. The illustrations of surgical treatises, on the other hand, had to depict *something never shown before*. So far Sudhoff's thesis. The relevance of his observations to our study of representations of Caesarean birth—which is in the domain of surgery—can be described preliminarily as follows: since no iconographic patterns for this event were available, the illustrators had to find "something new," and they found it not in books but through the more or less reliable contemporary testimony of people who had observed such scenes. This crucial point is confirmed by the comparison of the Caesarean scenes with other scenes accompanying them in those manuscripts that show a compartmental arrangement: these other scenes (coronations, battles, and council scenes) follow established patterns and resemble each other closely in various manuscripts. By contrast, the Caesarean birth scenes show a great variety in detail and composition. Let us retain one further important consequence of Sudhoff's reflections: the tension between tradition and new direct observation, which was one of the hallmarks of medieval medicine, was—at least in the domain of surgical illustration—resolved in favor of the latter.

Obstetrical and Gynecological Illustrations

Normal childbirth was, of course, not a surgical procedure. Consequently, its iconography follows a line of development different from that of surgery. The representations of births in the Middle Ages fall into two traditions: the antique medical one, reflecting ancient obstetrical practices, and the stylized Christian one, exemplified by the Nativity.[23] One of the most famous examples of the first tradition is a birth scene on folio 102r of Codex 93 in the National Library in Vienna.[24] This thirteenth-century illustration from the pseudo-Apuleian *Herbarium* is based on an antique model from about 550 A.D. and thus allows us to look back over many centuries into a birth chamber.[25] The fully dressed pregnant woman is seated on a birth stool with her knees apart. Four female attendants are grouped around her. Three of them support her back and shoulders while the fourth kneels to her left and holds a coriander sprig near the expectant mother's thigh. We learn from the text that the *herba coriandrum* hastens the birth.[26] It is interesting that even though the pseudo-Apuleian text offers no details on the birth itself, the grouping of the attendants and their actions accurately reflect Soranus's instructions to midwives.[27] Thus this birth scene independently illustrates a text that at this point is centuries old and does not even appear in this particular manuscript. The practices described and popularized in Soranus's *Gynecology* and its adaptations clearly had become an integral part of medieval medical and artistic thought.

This illustration, unlike many others, survived the Arabic transmission of antique medical texts, which was, as Sudhoff points out, incomplete because of religious proscriptions against representing the human body.[28] It is difficult to evaluate how absolute these proscriptions were. According to Herrlinger, the Arabic hostility toward images has been much exaggerated.[29] Apparently there were some realistic representations from the domains of surgery and obstetrics, but little research has been done in this field.[30] In any case, a birth is shown in a fourteenth-century Latin manuscript of Abulcasis's *Chirurgie,* where the illustrator made a misguided attempt at realism: he wanted to show the birth of twins, and consequently he painted two tiny heads, emerging at the same time from the birth canal—clearly a physical impossibility.[31] In the thirteenth-century Sarajevo *Haggadah,* Rebecca gives birth to her twins at the same time:[32] a striking parallel between a medical and a nonmedical miniature. Clearly, for some illuminators the dramatic aspects of showing the birth of twins were more important than medical accuracy.

Realistic images of childbirth are rare in medical manuscripts. Schematic representations of the uterus (with or without fetuses) or of pregnant women are more common. A ninth-century manuscript of Moschion's sixth-century adaptation of Soranus's *Gynecology,* for example, belongs to a special group of late antique clinical illustrations of the uterus.[33] A rather stunning group of "transparent" pregnant women adorns the margins and initials in a fourteenth-century manuscript of Albertus Magnus's *De animalibus.*[34] The number of fetuses carried by these women ranges from one, in a relatively small female figure, to twenty-four, in a giantess awkwardly occupying the right margin. "Transparent women" also appear in nonmedical representations: a number of fourteenth-century illustrations of the Visitation show the holy infants in the chest cavities of both Saint Elizabeth and the Virgin Mary.[35] In a wooden sculpture from 1320, the artist first cut holes into Mary's and Saint Elizabeth's chests, inserted the children and then closed the cavities with rock crystal.[36] A variation on the "transparent woman" is the depiction of Ecclesia in the fourteenth-century work of Opicinus de Canistris.[37] The iconography of the Virgin had influenced the representation of the church as a woman who would sometimes hold a child in her arms. Opicinus adds a medical element to this image: in addition to the child held by Ecclesia a naked infant is suspended upside down in front of her stomach, a design which seems to suggest pregnancy and imminent birth.

Fetal positions are also illustrated in many manuscripts, notably in texts of the Trotula tradition and in (later) manuals for midwives.[38] These schematic images were probably thought to be more useful to midwives than representations of actual births. The few medieval medical illustrations showing a normal birth in progress depended almost entirely on antique models.

In the nonmedical iconographic tradition of childbirth the oldest birth scene is probably that of a funeral stele of approximately the eighth century B.C.[39] This stele commemorated a mother's death in childbirth, a sad testimony to an ancient woman's fate. A more positive image can be found on a Corinthian vase that shows a successful birth in progress.[40]

Illuminated bibles are one of the best sources for nonmedical birth scenes; a stylized version of the birth of Christ developed early and became dominant for the depiction of most biblical births. More realistic scenes, such as the birth of Jacob and Esau in the seventh-century Ash-burnham Pentateuch and a birth in the fourteenth-century *Wenzelsbibel,* are noteworthy exceptions.[41] The representation of Rebecca in the Pen-tateuch, as she is being supported by female attendants, is in the same tradition as the scene in Vienna Codex 93 described above. The similarity between the two images, as well as between the images of the birth of twins and the "transparent women" mentioned above, illustrates the difficulty—or even the impossibility—of completely separating the med-ical from the nonmedical iconographic tradition. The birth of Alexander the Great, for example, in a fourteenth-century nonmedical manuscript (of the *Roman d'Alexandre*), contains details otherwise found in medical illustrations, especially the propping up of the mother by several atten-dants.[42] This particular motif is one of the important links between ancient obstetrical traditions as they are known from texts and as they can be seen in pictorial representations.

An extremely rare depiction of the birth of Christ that shows the influence of profane art appears in a late-thirteenth-century Florentine manuscript.[43] The *Stützmotiv* is used here even though the child is already born. The image thus combines the two important traditions for birth scenes: the antique medical tradition, which focuses on the birth as process, and the Christian tradition, which focuses on the birth as a state, that is, on the moment *after* the actual birth.

The tradition of representing a birth as "the moment after" prevailed, as becomes clear in Müllerheim's study of the birth chamber in art: his 138 illustrations show almost exclusively "religious" births (of Jesus, Mary, and John) and always as a scene after the birth itself.[44] In most of these images the mother lies in bed; usually she is fully dressed, but occasionally she seems to be naked but covered up.[45] A fire is kept going to warm the infant and its clothes; a bath is prepared and often the midwife or an attendant is bathing the newborn. Accessories, such as furniture, dishes, and bed clothes, vary, depending on the date of the illustration. This version of the Nativity lost some of its popularity after the fourteenth century. A new pattern emerged, focusing on the Virgin kneeling in front of the manger, her hands folded in prayer and adoration of the newborn Jesus.[46] The idea of birth as such is nonexistent in these pictures, and consequently illustrations of the Nativity are not the best sources for the study of medieval birth. The older pattern of the mother lying in bed with the infant by her side was perpetuated in representations of the birth of the Virgin, but it too became schematic and removed from obstetrical reality. Given this development toward schematization and given the strength of the iconographic tradition of the Nativity, our representations of Caesarean births take on special importance: they are not dependent on an obvious model; they do not all follow the same pattern and can consequently give us a more differentiated view of medieval birth.

TEXT AND IMAGE

How did the illustrators of medieval medical texts know what to depict? Did they read the passages they illustrated or did they merely provide general illustrations? Let us look at some examples.

In a fifteenth-century manuscript of Bartholomeus Anglicus's thirteenth-century encyclopedia *De proprietatibus rerum,* an extremely popular work, the illustration introducing a section on headache remedies shows not the herbs used in such remedies but rather what Imbault-Huart describes as a "raccourci complet de la médecine médiévale," that is, a surgeon doing a uroscopy by his patient's bedside and a pharmacy displaying shelves of various drugs; the pharmacist is weighing ingredients on a scale.[47] The illustrator clearly reproduced general images of what he knew of medieval medicine. An illustration in a late-thirteenth-century manuscript of Aldobrandina di Siena's *Li Livres dou santé* does not reflect the text either. As Jones points out, the young man dangling his feet in the water while waiting for leeches to attach themselves was a whimsy of the illustrator.[48] The text indicates that leeches were collected by doctors, stored in jars, and applied to patients indoors. But in most manuscripts a logical relationship between text and image exists. This does not necessarily mean that the illuminator had to read the text; instructions written in the margins of manuscripts indicate that someone read the text and then decided on the type of illumination it required. This information was transmitted to the artist via the marginal notes.

Sometimes, however, the scribe, not a specialized illuminator, was responsible for the illustrations. A good example is a manuscript of John of Arderne's *Speculum flebotomiae* (fig. 1).[49] On folio 94r the surgeon describes an emergency operation he performed on a three-day-old infant whose head had suffered through a protracted birth. When he explains exactly where he made the incision with a razor (in order to relieve pressure on the cranium), he refers to the illustration by saying "sicut hic depingitur" (as it is depicted here). The rather inept but charming image thus serves as an important visual aid to the text.

Henri de Mondeville supposedly used medical illustrations as well as practical demonstrations in his teaching. Thus, in manuscripts of his *Chirurgie,* there is a clear interdependency of text and image.[50] One of the most famous surgical manuscripts, the above-mentioned Sloane 1977, also illustrates the text by using schematic, but nevertheless useful, pictures that sometimes show isolated surgical interventions and at other times a whole operation from beginning to end.[51]

The ambiguity of the relationship between text and image also extended to illustrations of surgical instruments. There was a rich tradition, especially in Arabic manuscripts, in the depiction of these instruments, some of which will appear in representations of Caesarean births. Unlike scenes involving the human body, the representation of surgical instruments continued in an unbroken line from antiquity through the Arabic tradition to medieval Europe. In some cases, the illustrators copied their predecessors so exactly that they also repeated their mistakes. A rather amusing example is the depiction of a vaginal speculum in a fourteenth-century manuscript of the Latin translation of Abulcasis where "the artist has missed the mechanical point altogether."[52] The screw meant to open the two blades of the speculum has taken on a curious flowerlike appearance; a kite-shaped appendix on the right is supposed to be a separate scalpel. The textual corruption evident in so many medieval (medical and nonmedical) manuscripts thus finds its counterpart in the corruption of the iconographic transmission. Texts and images clearly encountered similar problems in their travels through the centuries.

The iconography of childbirth represents a special case, as it seems to have developed independently from any textual tradition of obstetrics. Most obstetric texts, if they have any illustrations at all, restrict themselves to schematic drawings of fetal positions. More explicit images of childbirth in medical manuscripts often have no direct relation to the text they accompany, as we saw for the pseudo-Apuleian *Herbarium,* which shows a splendid realistic birth scene in the section on the herb coriander. Nonmedical manuscripts, on the other hand, such as the Bible, the *Roman d'Alexandre,* and the *Faits des Romains,* contain medically accurate birth scenes even though the texts often give only the vaguest information on the birth as such. Illustrators seemed more inclined to show the birth of a specific hero or biblical character than childbirth per se (or perhaps were paid to do so). In almost every instance, the birth scenes can be situated in an iconographic tradition, often relying on antique models. The case is quite different for Caesarean births: unlike other birth scenes, scenes of Caesarean births do not follow an iconographic tradition, because none existed.

Another reason for the relatively infrequent illustration of childbirth in medical manuscripts may be the small role obstetrics played in the university curriculum and surgical education. The great medical and surgical handbooks concentrated on illustrating those procedures their readers were likely to perform themselves.

Thus the iconography of childbirth developed into a paradox: the most accurate obstetrical illustrations were those found outside of medical manuscripts. The readers of copies and translations of ancient historical texts or of the Bible were much more likely to encounter images of childbirth than those readers studying medical works.

WOMEN IN MEDICAL ILLUSTRATIONS

Women were depicted in a variety of roles in medical illustrations.[53] The best known among the women shown as healers was the (possibly legendary) Trotula of Salerno. In Wellcome manuscript 544 she "is holding an orb in her left hand signifying that she is an 'empress' among midwives."[54] Midwives are of course common in Nativity scenes, where their function is mostly to hold or bathe the infant. But women also have other healing functions. In a Flemish manuscript of 1470, we see a bearded patient in bed while a woman sits on a stool in front of the hearth; she is stirring something—most likely an herbal concoction—in a pot; she is probably following a recipe from the book that is lying open on her lap. Her headdress identifies her as a healer.[55] In an illustration from a fifteenth-century psalter, a nurse is feeding a sick man; a fourteenth-century manuscript of the *Tacuinum sanitatis* shows a woman apothecary preparing medicine in a pharmacy.[56] A woman can be seen performing one of the minor surgical functions, bloodletting by cupping, in a fifteenth-century English manuscript.[57] Thus women were represented in a number of healing functions, especially as midwives, of course.[58] Still, it is in the scenes of Caesarean birth that women's capacities for quick, decisive action and surgical skills are evoked most vividly. Most other representations of women in medicine emphasize tranquil concern and care for patients or pupils.

The usefulness of the types of illustrations just described to the historian of medieval medicine has been debated. Eugen Holländer, in his *Medizin in der Klassischen Malerei* (Medicine in classical painting) claims that "representations of this kind [that is, scenes of births] are of only limited interest because painters and illustrators never had the opportunity to be present at such a scene."[59] Holländer has reservations particularly about images of Caesarean birth. But as he uses only one isolated sixteenth-century example, his remarks can hardly be accepted as a sound critical approach.[60] Some of the birth scenes discussed above, such as the ones in Vienna Codex 93 or the Ashburnham Pentateuch, reflect ancient medical teaching of which more than a few traces were left in medieval Europe. Other, later, images, such as the woodcuts for Roesslin's or Rueff's treatises, directly illustrate the advice given in the text. The major nonmedical group of birth scenes, the Nativity and the births of Mary and Saint John, it is true, are of more interest to historians of the birth chamber than to the medical historian. Once again, therefore, the value of the series of images in this book becomes obvious: twenty-six representations of midwives and surgeons performing the same operation are a sufficient sample for an examination not only of the operation itself but also of its participants.

MIDWIVES AND SURGEONS IN IMAGES OF
CAESAREAN BIRTHS

Midwives at Work

The series of birth scenes I will now consider in detail chronicles the beginning of one of the most important transformations for medieval and early modern medicine: the slow incursion of men into the fields of obstetrics and gynecology. The atmosphere in these scenes is quite different from that of the Nativity, since Caesarean birth allows for a depiction of birth as process; it does not require an illustrator to show the normal position of a woman during birth, a position that was considered immodest, and yet it gave artists the opportunity to depict nude bodies. Thus, for the art historian, the illustrations could prove useful as sources for the representation of the nude female body as well as of newborn babies in medieval art. I will concentrate on the actual operation and on the representation of gender roles, however.

The oldest illustration of the group (fig. 4) dates from the late thirteenth century. It is thus almost contemporaneous with the appearance of the first surgical text describing the operation, Bernard of Gordon's *Lilium* (1305), not as an illustration of this text but as a representation of Julius Caesar's birth in a vernacular manuscript of Roman history, the *Faits des Romains*.

On the left in figure 4 the adult Caesar is holding a council; on the right his birth takes place under dramatic circumstances. The mother's naked body, covered by a sheet from the waist down, reclines on a kind of couch. Her eyes are closed, her mouth is open, her right arm supports her upper body. Her left side is propped up by one of the attendants, while the operating midwife holds the mother's left arm by the wrist to move it out of the way. The two women involved in the actual operation are wearing a type of headdress different from that of the other three women; they are undoubtedly midwives, whereas the others may be friends, neighbors, or family members. The midwife on the right bends over so much that her back is horizontal, an attitude that conveys great urgency and concentration. She is making a left lateral incision with a curved razor above the mother's navel. The other midwife pulls out the disproportionately large child by both hands. The little Caesar has emerged just about halfway. He has lots of curly hair and a rather mature expression on his face—none of the crumpled-up wrinkles of a real newborn here. As for

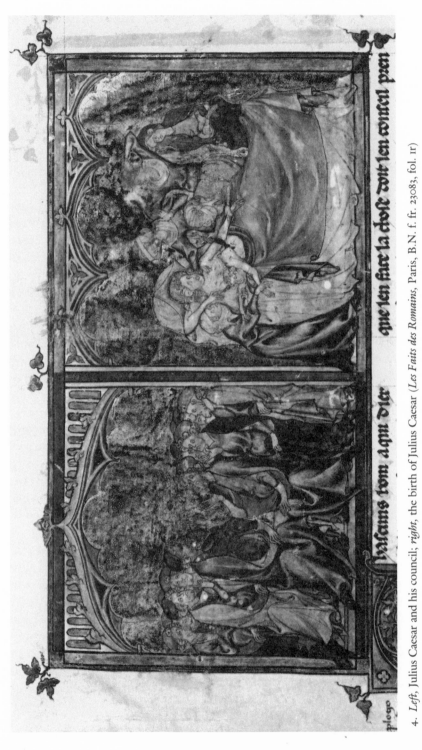

4. *Left*, Julius Caesar and his council; *right*, the birth of Julius Caesar (*Les Faits des Romains*), Paris, B.N. f. fr. 23083, fol. 1r

the mother, it is not quite clear from her looks whether she is alive or dead, although the touching gestures of mourning and lamentation on the part of the attendants—the one in the center seems to be tearing out her hair—suggest that Caesar's mother has in fact died.

The six women form a solid group and yet dramatic energy is released through the diagonal line formed by the surgical razor and the child. We are clearly in the middle of a desperate situation where lives are at stake.

For the composition of this scene the artist could consult the text of the *Faits,* from which he could gather that "the cutting of the belly" was to be shown.[61] The vagueness of the French term *ventre* undoubtedly accounts for the artist's error in placing the uterus above the navel. The only other bit of concrete information was that "Caesar had a lot of hair," a characteristic faithfully rendered in this picture.

Some illustrators had additional clues as to what to depict in the scene of Caesar's birth. It is extremely fortunate that one example of marginal instructions to the illustrator has survived. In manuscript Garrett 128 (fig. 3), which dates from the late fourteenth century, we read in the left margin on folio 144r: "Famez q*ui* ouvre le ventre d'une fame a couteus et e*n* traient un enfant qui a g*rans* cheveus" (a woman who opens the belly of a woman with a knife and pulls out a child who has a lot of hair). These instructions are rather scanty, but they contain some details not found in the *Faits:* that the incision is to be made with a knife and that one "pulls out" the child. And indeed, the small image that forms the historiated initial "C" contains all the elements referred to in the marginal instructions. The large median incision differs from the one in figure 4, but the child is just as oversize and the mother's right arm is lifted up in a similar way. Here, however, she is not covered by a blanket and the same midwife who made the incision also pulls out the child. The author of the marginal instructions, possibly the "conceptualizer" of the manuscript, specified that a woman (midwife) was to be shown as performing the operation, undoubtedly a reflection of contemporary practice.[62]

Let us now look at illustrations in a group of (probably Parisian) manuscripts from the mid-fourteenth century: figures 5, 6, and 7. In figures 5 and 6 the important events of Caesar's life are chronicled in groups of four illuminations: his birth, Caesar receiving petitioners, and his twofold coronation as "bishop" and emperor. The manuscript of figure 7 replaces the two scenes on the right with Caesar's divorce and a battle. Whereas architectural motifs divide the illuminations in figures 5 and 6, polylobes frame the image in figure 7. Despite these differences the

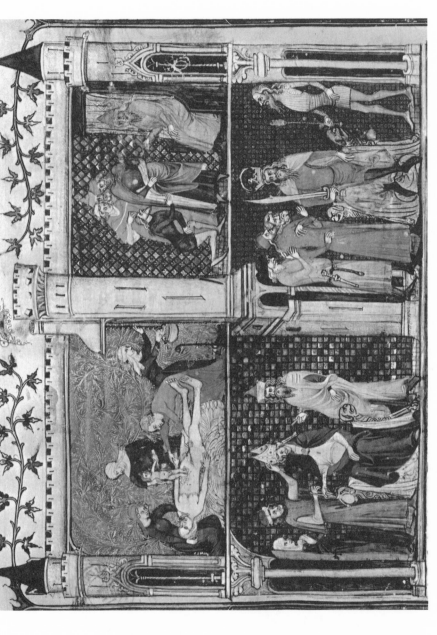

5. *Upper left*, the birth of Julius Caesar; *right*, Caesar and a suppliant. *Lower left*, Caesar as bishop; *right*, Caesar as emperor (*Les Faits des Romans*, Paris, B.N. n. acq. fr. 3576, fol. 197r)

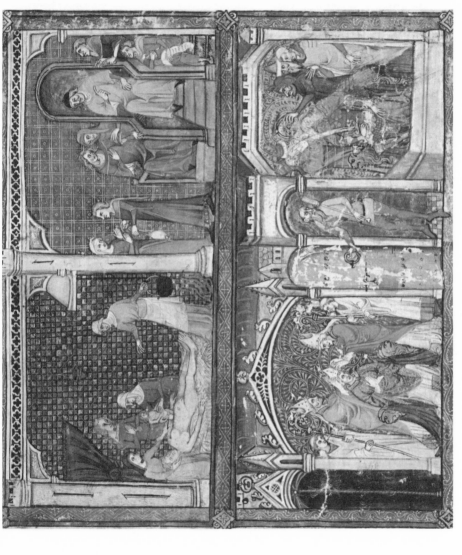

6. *Upper left*, the birth of Julius Caesar; *right*, Caesar giving an audience. *Lower left*, Caesar's coronation as bishop and, *right*, as emperor (*Les Faits des Romains*, Paris, B.N. f. fr. 246, fol. 158r)

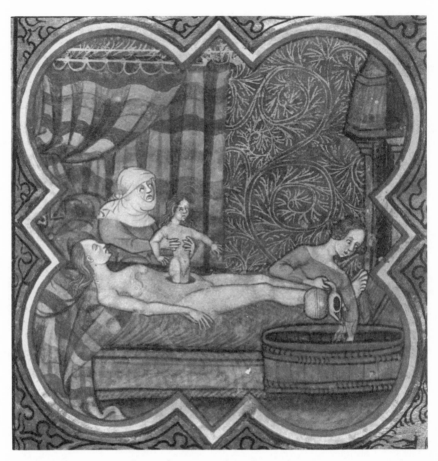

7. The birth of Julius Caesar (*Les Faits des Romains*, London, British Library, Royal MS G 16 VII, fol. 219r)

birth scenes themselves all show the same basic arrangement: the mother, obviously dead, is stretched out naked from left to right on a low couch. In figures 5 and 7, the abdominal opening is located in the center of the mother's body and is clearly visible. The operation is already over and one of the midwives is pulling out a curly-haired infant. In figure 5 the illustrator included some realistic features: in the large, centrally placed incision some "organs" can be discerned, drawn in a manner reminiscent of the intestines in the first representations of autopsies.[63] In a significant attempt at medical realism the artist shows one woman holding open the mouth of the mother, while another steadies the mother's body with her right hand; her left hand possibly holds open the entrance to the mother's vagina. We recall that these two measures were supposed to prevent the suffocation of the fetus.

This group of illustrations falls into the period of the publication of Guy de Chauliac's *Grande chirurgie,* where he mentions both the recommended place for the incision and the "habit of ignorant women" to hold open the mouth of a woman being delivered by Caesarean section. Like Guy's text, the illustrator's version of Caesarean birth thus reflects the medical lore of the time. Whether the artist obtained this information from a medical text or directly from medical practitioners is hard to determine. The logical division of labor among the women, the arrangement of the figures, the presence of such details as water being heated in the hearth, all suggest that the illuminators actually consulted midwives. They may have supplemented this information with medical texts, of course. For the earliest example (fig. 4), however, it is unlikely that the artist could have used any medical texts. Bernard of Gordon's *Lilium,* the first-known treatise to mention Caesarean birth, was not available until 1305, and even then it was probably not widely diffused, certainly not outside of university circles. Consequently there must have been some contact between illustrators and medical practitioners. In any case, it is remarkable that the first—and only—image that shows the holding open of the mother's mouth, should have been produced almost contemporaneously with Guy's text.

The three illustrations we have been discussing resemble each other closely and yet some of the details are different: figure 7 shows one midwife and one helper, whereas in figure 5 four women are concentrating on the business of the operation and the subsequent care of the infant. But as in figure 6, only two of the women are wearing the headdress characteristic of midwives in this period. The others, undoubtedly instructed by the midwives, are helpers. Such helpers would be present at most births; in fact, if a birth promised to be normal, some women, especially in rural areas, never called in a midwife and relied instead on relatives and neighbors.[64] It is remarkable, then, that in figures 5 and 6 a team of two midwives is at work. Since the workload of a midwife could reach up to three hundred births a year, the presence of two midwives at a single birth indicates the importance—and the anticipated difficulties—of Caesarean delivery.[65]

In addition to physical assistance, a midwife also needed spiritual support in the critical situation of a pregnant woman's impending death.

She not only had to make a decision on whether to perform the operation, she also had to act extremely quickly: she had to make the incision, pull out the child, and baptize the infant if it looked weak. The risks involved in this operation were manifold, and not the least was the danger for the midwife of being accused of bungling or, worse, of deliberately killing the newborn. Since in most Caesareans neither the mother nor the infant survived, midwives must have welcomed witnesses, and especially professional witnesses, in order to be able to clear their record in the case of accusations.[66] Also, fifteenth-century regulations explicitly instructed midwives to call in another midwife for difficult or risky births.[67]

The midwives in these three illustrations are obviously competent, as they carry out a well-orchestrated procedure that also involves the helpers in useful ways. The gestures of mourning and despair, so prevalent in figure 4, are limited in this group of images to a single woman in figure 6, who stands with folded hands in a contemplative stance. The other women are all actively engaged in attending to mother and child. The denigration of the midwives' competence, of which we saw an example in Guy de Chauliac's text, certainly did not find its way into these images.

There is a certain starkness to these scenes. The accessories are reduced to a minimum, the furniture is stylized: a covered couch, maybe some draperies.[68] The absence of distracting details, of course, heightens the drama of the action and contrasts quite sharply with the elaborate interior scenes of the later (fifteenth-century) group of Caesarean births. Also, the later representations of Caesar's birth often stand alone and thus emphasize the birth much more than those images where the birth scene forms part of a compartmentalized miniature illustrating the major events in Caesar's life. Since men play a much more important role in these later images, we will have to ask ourselves what could have prompted this different iconographic schema. But let us first return to the group at hand.

The other scenes in figures 5, 6, and 7 show coronations (both secular and ecclesiastic) and councils. Figure 4, as well, features a council scene on the left. The manuscript of figure 8 provides the richest series of images: in addition to Caesar's birth, it features the plotting followers of Catilina engaged in a conversation; Caesar's coronation; two conquests of towns; and Caesar's assassination. Another manuscript, Condé 726, adds two new elements on folio 175r: Caesar's triumph and his contemplation of the statue of Alexander the Great.[69] Most frequently, then, Caesar's birth forms part of a whole series of images illustrating his life.

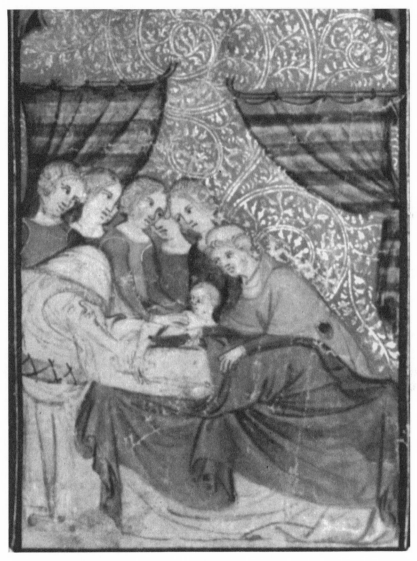

8. The birth of Julius Caesar (*Les Faits des Romains*, Copenhagen, Kongelige Bibliotek, MS Thott 431, fol. 224r)

His childhood and youth are neglected, undoubtedly because that part was missing from Suetonius's *The Twelve Caesars*. Information on his birth came from Isidore of-Seville's *Etymologies*. Although, traditionally, Caesarean birth was considered a miracle foretelling a hero's great destiny, the author of the *Faits des Romains* did not even devote a whole paragraph to Caesar's birth and did not attach any prophecies to this event. It is therefore all the more remarkable how frequently and in what great detail his entrance into the world was depicted. But it was by the manner of his birth, of course, that he—at least in the opinion of medieval scholars—gained his famous name. Whether the etymological derivation from *caesus* (cut) or from *caesaries* (hair) was favored, in either case his birth explained his name and was therefore a vital scene.

In the illustrations that show both his secular and ecclesiastical coronation we see two quite different Caesars, modeled on the "types" of the bishop and the emperor: as the former, Caesar is clean-shaven and has short hair; as the latter, he sports a full beard and an impressive mane of hair. If only the coronation as bishop is represented, it also conforms to the pattern of the beardless and shorthaired church dignitary. It is extremely important to notice the difference between these scenes and the birth scenes: the coronations and council scenes all follow a familiar schema; after all, these were scenes very frequently shown in historical and religious manuscripts. The birth scenes, on the other hand, show great variation even if they appear in the same compartmentalized miniature as a traditional coronation. The scenes around figure 8, for example, represent an ecclesiastical coronation identical to those in figures 5, 6, 7, and 9, and yet the Caesarean birth in figure 8 is completely different from the rest: the mother is draped in various cloths, and the woman who operates does not wear the characteristic headdress but rather the type of hairdo that can also be found in figure 10. Other resemblances between figures 8 and 10 include the position of the attendant(s) and of the (dead) mother, the attitude of the operating woman, and the location of the incision. Note, however, the oversized surgical knife in figure 10: a truly frightening sight. Did the illuminator aim for high drama or was he simply misinformed as to the size of such a knife?

It is possible that female surgeons rather than midwives are performing the operation in figures 8, 9, and 10. Figure 9 is especially suggestive of this possibility because a midwife is also present; the illustrator was aware of a midwife's appropriate costume and shows her ready to receive the

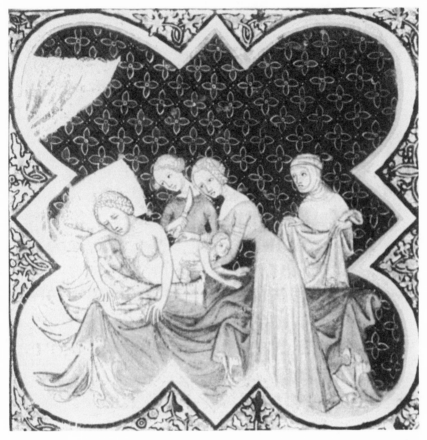

9. The birth of Julius Caesar (*Les Faits des Romains,* MS in the Schöyen Collection, fol. 199r)

newborn in a large white sheet.[70] The distinction in dress between the two women thus probably indicates their different professions: midwife and "surgeoness."[71]

So far we have seen mostly scenes in which the mother was dead or moribund. In figures 5, 6, and 7 the mother's body looks corpselike; stretched out lifelessly, her body is being manipulated by the midwives and attendants. In figures 4, 9, and 10 the mother's eyes are closed and she seems to have fainted. Her body is in a semirecumbent position. However, in at least two of the illustrations the mother looks alive: in figure 2, her eyes are open even though she does not look at the child. In one manuscript (Condé 726, fol. 175r), the mother looks alive and content.

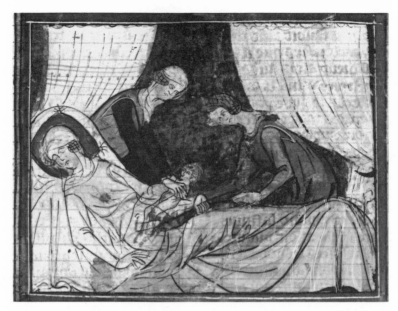

10. The birth of Julius Caesar (*Les Faits des Romains,* Brussels, Bibliothèque Royale, MS 9104–9105, fol. 218r)

She supports her head with her right hand while with her left hand she cheerfully points to an enormous (adult-size) baby standing on her left knee. A figure whose gender cannot be determined, dressed in a lavender colored gown, lends some support to the "baby."

Such an unlikely scene may have reflected the views of some medieval chroniclers who were well aware of the discrepancy between the legend of Caesar's birth by abdominal delivery (known to be fatal to the mother) and Caesar's mentioning his mother as still being alive during his conquest of Gaul. Thus some illustrators wanted to reconcile the story of the survival of Caesar's mother with the depiction of a Caesarean birth and consequently ended up with a scene that did not quite correspond to the medieval medical experience. Each illustrator had to compose his own version of the "truth." Most of them chose to be true to obstetrical reality, but others decided differently. The result was a wide variety of birth scenes, which is much more valuable to us than conformity to any one pattern could have been.

Of all the illustrations of the early group, figure 2 is the only one that does not show the actual operation. It is also the only one that contains two successive moments in one image (a common medieval device); first, the naked curly-haired baby is being lifted from his mother's lap by two attendants (who, incidentally, look exactly like the mother), and then, on the right, the newborn is wrapped in swaddling clothes like a little mummy. The mother, who is reclining fully dressed on a draped low couch, shows no direct traces of a Caesarean birth—or a normal birth, for that matter. She may be weakened, however, for her attitude is listless and she does not watch her newborn son.

All the other early manuscripts show the performance of the operation and thus present us with a vivid picture of a medieval medical procedure. We have already mentioned the great variety of the birth scenes. Nevertheless, iconographic models for the depiction of the operation have been suggested. Fritz Weindler reproduced two illustrations from Josef Kirchner's book on the representation of Adam and Eve: Eve "born" from Adam's side is supposed to have supplied the iconographic scheme for a Caesarean birth.[72] A careful examination of all these early illustrations, however, reveals only a single example that corresponds somewhat to the creation of Eve: figure 9; all the others do not really show a birth from the flank, nor do they follow a single pattern. They have only one thing in common: they make an attempt to show a realistic medical scene.

With the notable exception of figure 10, in most of the illustrations the instrument used for the operation is the correct one, a surgical razor; the incision is sometimes misplaced, but at other times it is in a logical place; the midwives, surgeonesses, and attendants all show a sense of purpose and a reasonable division of labor. Even though not one of the pictures shows the umbilical cord, they do not come out of the realm of fantasy. They show the domestic domain of giving birth, a dramatic birth, it is true, but clearly one that women could handle without male assistance or interference.

The entire earlier group of illustrations (up to about 1400) shows only midwives at work. In the later group a dramatic change takes place: women are relegated to the status of helpmates while male surgeons perform Caesarean sections. Only direct testimony from the participants in the operation can account for such a clear-cut transformation, especially as the gender of the personnel is one of the very few uniform features within each group. Except for this one extremely significant uniformity, the images show a great diversity in composition, that is, even though most illustrators use identical pictorial elements, they arrange them in a variety of different ways. In other words, the illustrators all knew what to depict in their images but were not bound by a common model or an iconographic schema.

Male Surgeons at Work

In the second group of images of Caesarean birth, those produced in the fifteenth century, everything changes—the nature of the birth, the decor, the attendants. We are now dealing with an official royal birth that has been taken over by male surgeons and has lost the intimate character of the earlier examples.[73] Could it be that the idea of portraying a royal birth, not a change in the practice of Caesareans, was responsible for the new type of medical personnel? I do not believe so. Royal births were attended by male practitioners much earlier, as Edward J. Kealy has shown.[74] Thus a male presence at such births was not a fifteenth-century innovation. The appearance of male surgeons in scenes of Caesarean birth therefore must be attributed to a change in the practice of that particular operation.

Of course, it was not only medical reality that brought about artistic changes. With the fifteenth century we enter an age of new splendor and new techniques in manuscript illumination. Most of the examples of the second group come from either Flemish or Burgundian workshops, the centers of fifteenth-century illumination. The text of the *Faits des Romains* saw a last great revival of its popularity in the Burgundy of Charles the Bold, and many of the late manuscripts of the *Faits* were copied during his lifetime and for some time afterward. But there are also new and different texts that are accompanied by illustrations of Caesar's birth: Jean Mansel's *Histoires romaines* (1454) and Jean du Chesnes's translation of Caesar's *Commentaries* (after 1474).[75] Both texts used the *Faits* for the account of Caesar's birth, so that the fifteenth-century illustrators had the same scanty textual base for the representation of Caesar's birth as the artists of the preceding centuries. But they, too, seem to have had other sources of information about the operation: they uniformly depict male surgeons, a transformation from the fourteenth century of which they must have learned from contemporary witnesses. The medical details such as the location of the incision are, in most cases, rendered accurately. The atmosphere is that of an official birth; the surroundings have become more splendid. But the suffering of the dead or dying mother is as intense

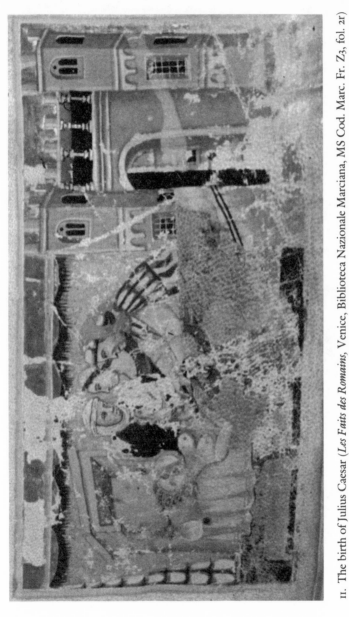

11. The birth of Julius Caesar (*Les Faits des Romains*, Venice, Biblioteca Nazionale Marciana, MS Cod. Marc. Fr. Z3, fol. 2r)

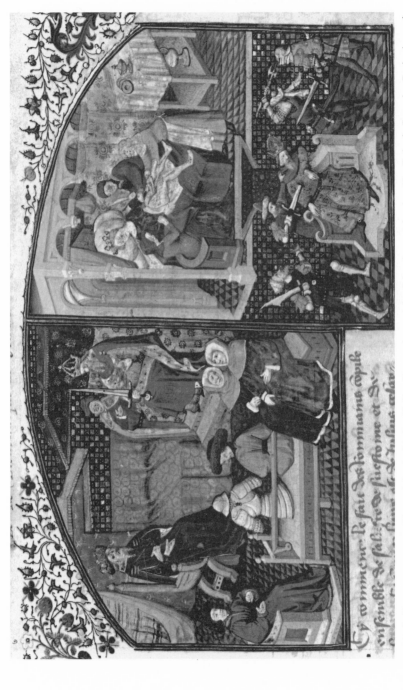

12. *Left*, Caesar as emperor. *Upper right*, the birth of Julius Caesar; *lower right*, Caesar's assassination (*Les Faits des Romains*, Paris, Arsenal, MS 5186, fol. 1r)

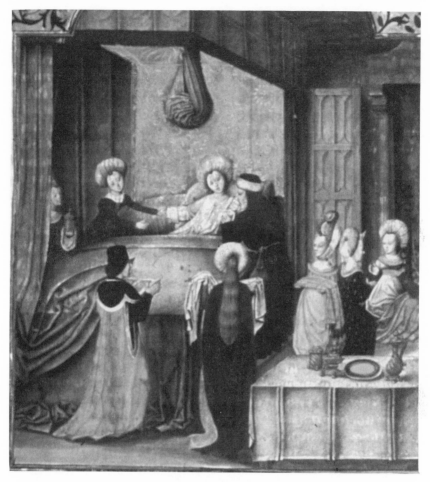

13. The birth of Julius Caesar (*Les Faits des Romains*, London, British Library, Royal MS 17 F II, fol. 9r)

as in the earlier pictures. In the fifteenth-century group, only two of the women can possibly be said to be alive: those in figures 13 and 14.

Of all the later birth scenes only two resemble each other: figures 15 and 16; the others show a striking variety—a renewed proof that the artists did not have a master model for the Caesarean operation. They had to create their own version of this obstetrical drama and must have done so by consulting medical practitioners.

One of the most violent representations of Caesar's birth can be found in figure 12. This manuscript has no further illuminations after folio 1, a

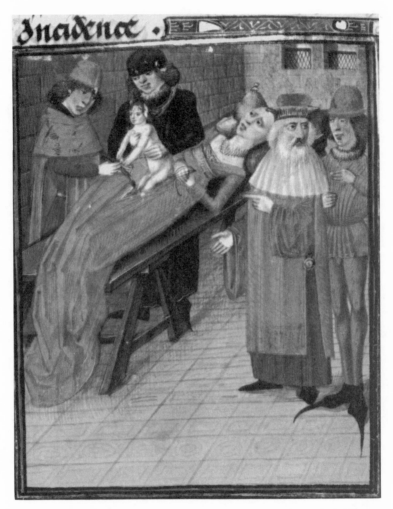

14. The birth of Julius Caesar (*Commentaires de César,* London, British Library, Royal MS 16 G VIII, fol. 32r)

sign that Caesar's entire life was thought to be encompassed by this initial group of illustrations: his birth; a council over which he presides, clad as emperor; and his assassination. The birth is placed directly above the murder scene; in both images a knife (or dagger) occupies a central position, as if to suggest that he who was born by the sword must also die by it.

This illumination has several unusual features: it is the only one in

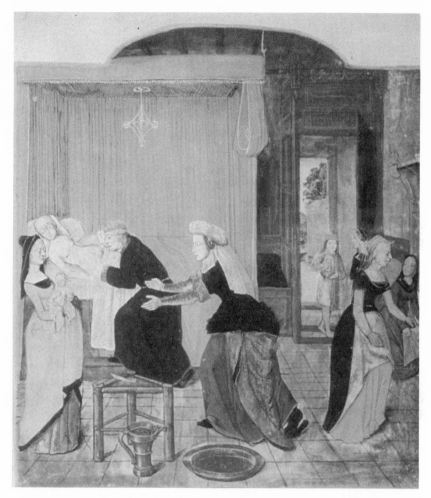

15. The birth of Julius Caesar (*Commentaires de César*, London, British Library, MS Egerton 1065, fol. 9r)

which the mother is wearing a crown and the only one in which the mother's body is nude from the waist down, rather than completely (corpselike) nude or covered up to the waist. The disarray of her clothes, more than anything else, indicates an emergency. The male surgeon, holding a slightly curved surgical razor in his right hand, has just made a long median incision along the *linea alba*. A haglike midwife pulls the newborn out of a gaping wound. The child, much smaller than those in the previous examples, has neither the perky looks nor the curly hair of

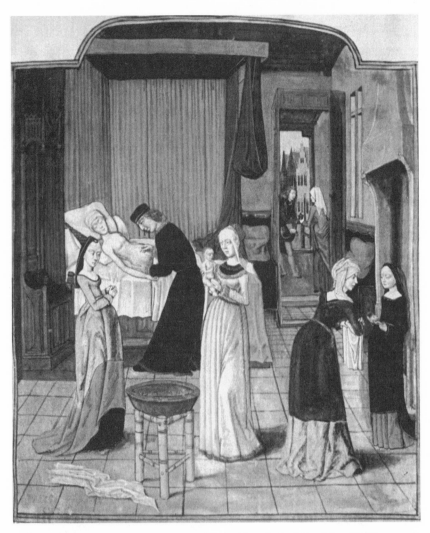

16. The birth of Julius Caesar (*Commentaires de César*, Oxford, Bodleian, MS Douce 208, fol. 1r)

his fourteenth-century predecessors. A female onlooker on the left seems to be pronouncing a prayer. The room where the operation takes place is much better defined than the birth chambers in the fourteenth-century manuscripts. There is a good attempt at perspective in the arched structure above the bed and in the table holding various golden vessels and implements. The table is covered with a precious cloth, and in the background we can see elegantly patterned curtains. These dignified surroundings contrast sharply with the bloody operation. Nothing is stylized here: the child is not pulled out ceremoniously through the mother's nightgown as in figure 13—here we see the incision, the blood, and the awkward position of the half-naked woman. This is surely one of the most moving of all our images.

In figure 12 the group of scenes of Caesar's life is still divided into compartments as in the fourteenth-century examples, but the division is not hermetic here: the upper part of Caesar's throne protrudes into the lower part of the birth chamber. As the fifteenth century progresses, the compartmentalized miniature is abandoned more and more, and different scenes begin to exist side by side in complicated architectural and natural landscapes.

Splendid examples of this new technique are figures 17 and 18. Figure 17, produced about 1460, is packed with action: Caesar's birth takes place on the left in a pillared structure that holds an elegant canopied bed. The lower right shows the cruel scene of the strangling of one of Catilina's accomplices. A battle scene occupies the space above, and on the upper right Caesar seems to be contemplating the statue of Alexander the Great, a wonderful rendering of a contemplative stance. Sailboats float on the horizon while the street in the center is populated by a small dog and a crane.[76] As in figure 12, the juxtaposition of two violent scenes—the bloody Caesarean operation and the strangling in the Tullianum—is most effective. In both pictures death is central, and yet the relative calm of the birth scene contrasts with while complementing the energetic movements of the strangling. The sense of urgency that could be felt in figure 12 is replaced here by a sad resignation, expressed in the mournful face of the surgeon and the praying gesture of the woman behind the bed. The mother, lying naked on a large bed, seems drained of all blood, which gushes forth from a long lateral incision on the right. The surgeon, recognizable as one of the higher class of surgeons by his long robe, carefully pulls a very large child out of the wound. As in all the other images, there is no trace of an umbilical cord. The woman on the right has prepared a sheet to receive the newborn. She is dressed rather elegantly in a red dress with a draped tunic slipped over it, a doughnutlike head ornament, and a necklace. This outfit suggests that she is not a midwife but rather one of the attendants of Caesar's mother. The woman on the left has a slightly simpler look and could be a midwife assisting the surgeon. The surgeon himself advertises his wealth and status through

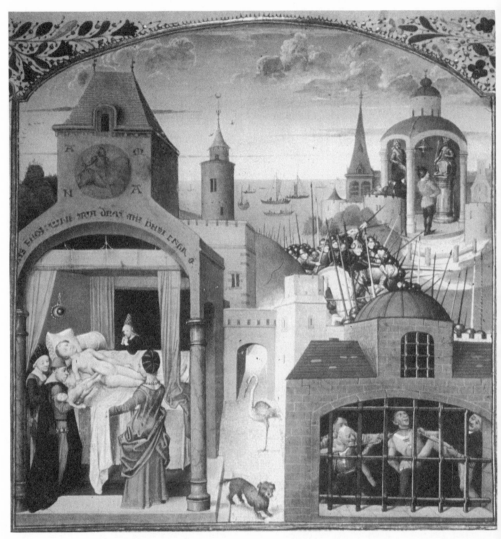

17. *Left,* the birth of Julius Caesar; in the background, a battle scene. *Upper right,* Caesar contemplating a statue of Alexander the Great. *Lower right,* a follower of Catalina being killed in the Tullianum (*Les Faits des Romains,* Paris, B.N. f. fr. 64, fol. 234r.)

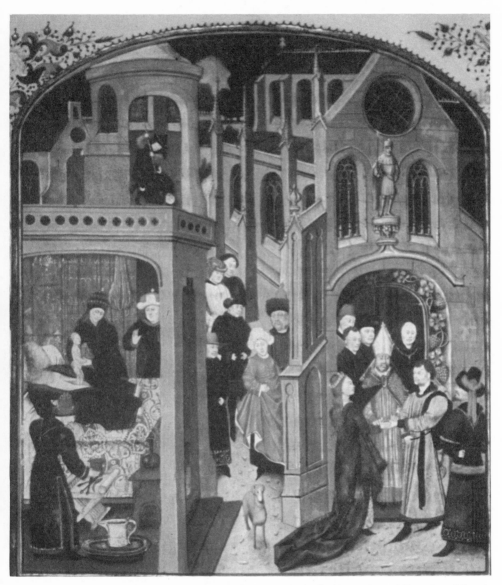

18. *Left,* the birth of Julius Caesar. Above, a murder. *Right,* Julius Caesar's wedding (Jean Mansel, *Histoires romaines,* Paris, Arsenal, MS 5088, fol. 43r)

the splendid blue cloak worn over his red robe and held together by a gold ornament: a subtle suggestion perhaps that at least the surgical part of obstetrics may have become lucrative enough to interest a surgeon of the class depicted here.[77]

A comparison of this illumination with the fourteenth-century examples reveals that the women have become marginal and passive. The energetic postures of the earlier midwives give way here to more static ones. In fact, the female figures provide the compositional frame for the central elements of the image: the mother and the male surgeon who are connected by the vertical line of the baby.

Whereas in figure 17 women play at least a marginal role, in figure 18 they are totally absent. The illustrator of this Flemish manuscript of Jean Mansel's *Histoires romaines* chose a composition not unlike that of figure 17 for his frontispiece. The birth takes place on the left in a well-defined architectural structure. On the right, a bishop blesses the union of Caesar and his bride at the entrance (rather than inside as in modern times) of a beautiful Gothic church. A dog, possibly a symbol of fidelity, is among the onlookers at the center. On the top left, a murder takes place (again Catilina's followers?), reaffirming the connection we had noted earlier between Caesar's birth and violence.

In the birth scene, all three participants are men, dressed in long robes. Despite the brocaded splendor of the bedroom we feel that we are in an operating room: on a stool the surgeon has laid out several instruments, including, on the right, the curved razor recommended for the operation by Guy de Chauliac. The man in the foreground holds some kind of a container and on the floor stands a water basin with a large golden pitcher in it. The mother is covered by a dark robe, except for the center of her body, where the garment is thrown open to allow for a median incision. The mother's face is unrecognizable: it was erased for some unknown reason. The surgeon, wearing a splendid headdress, tenderly and carefully removes the child from the wound. An impressed witness on the right observes the proceedings. The homely touches of the birth, such as a sheet held ready or a warm bath, are missing in this image. As in figure 17, the splendid robes, the magnificence of the birth chamber, and the male presence transform Caesar's birth into a royal birth—more a matter of state perhaps than a domestic, feminine affair.

The same atmosphere reigns in our next two examples: an illustration in manuscript Condé 770 (about 1480) and figure 19, from a Flemish manuscript of the second half of the fifteenth century. In both illustra-

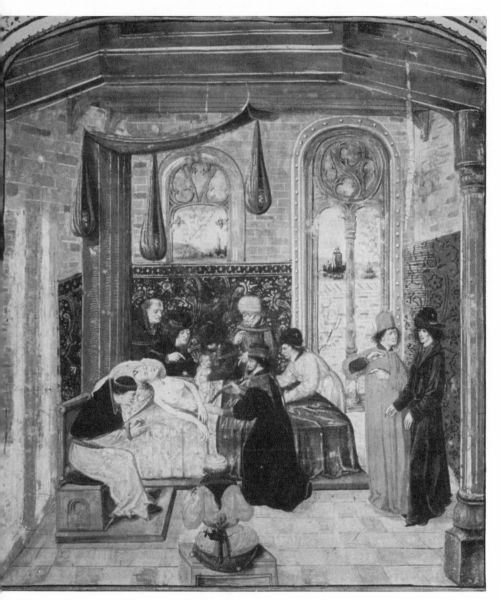

. The birth of Julius Caesar (*Les Faits des Romains,* Paris, B.N. f. fr. 20312 bis, fol. 1r)

tions an ecclesiastic participates in the scene; seated at the lower left, he lends a certain solemnity to the occasion. In the manuscript Condé 770 picture, the dead mother is stretched out on a bed while the surgeon, still holding up his knife, removes the child from an incision on her lower right thigh area. Several bearded counselors look on, while two women lament and cry on the right. Again, dogs can be found near the birth. Women appear only marginally and as passive onlookers.

In figure 19, no women are present. The operation is in progress: A bearded surgeon in a blue robe decorated with fur holds a long curved knife with which he has just made an incision on the lower right part of the mother's body. Blood is flowing from the wound; the mother has clearly died. Another bearded surgeon carefully lifts up the child. His gestures are of a tenderness seldom found in the depiction of medieval men.[78] A male attendant at the foot of the bed appears to hold ready a sheet. Except for the surgeons, all the men are clean-shaven, including the two ecclesiastics and the two men on the right, who seem to be discussing the operation. As in figure 14, where the operating table and the attitudes of the participants suggest a dissection, here the viewer's attention is drawn to the medical (possibly instructive) aspects of the operation rather than exclusively to the human drama. That is, the onlookers are not lamenting or praying but rather observing the procedure with a detached and professional eye.

Figure 19 has, with ten male participants, the largest personnel of any of the illustrations. Figure 13 comes close with two men and six women. Here, a burly-looking surgeon pulls a baby, for once tiny, from the folds of the mother's nightgown. A younger man, possibly a cleric, is reading from a book at the foot of the bed. One of the women holds up a sheet, others are bringing more. On the left, one of the attendants is offering a container (with drink?) that could be meant for the mother, who appears to be still alive. Consequently, we do not find here the detached medical interest evident in the previous example but rather a general air of solicitousness and concern, not only for the baby but for the mother as well.

This is also true for figures 15 and 16. The two illuminations resemble each other closely. In both of them the surgeons attend to the mother *after* the baby has been delivered, a new feature in these illustrations. While an attendant on the left is ready to hand the baby to a midwife, the surgeons seem to be suturing or at least closing the wound (along the *linea alba*). The curved surgical razor lies abandoned on a stool. The attention and special care that had been reserved for the newborn in our previous illustrations now also extend to the mother. For the first time the procedure of closing the wound is represented, an innovation that may have been prompted by medical developments, or at least by reports of such developments. For although, objectively speaking, nothing in the medical conditions of the operation had changed at that time to make truly successful Caesareans more likely, there had been *reports* of successful Caesarean operations in the fifteenth century; in 1411 a midwife was said to have delivered seven babies by Caesarean with both the mothers and the babies surviving.[79] The fifteenth century also saw male surgeons performing Caesareans, as we know from the testimony of Piero d'Argellata who, in his *Chirurgia,* described an operation he himself had performed. These changes in medical thought and practice are reflected in the illustrations shown here.

Although in a few of the earlier illustrations the mother looked alive, it is only in the later fifteenth-century representations that the artists emphasized the medical side of the mother's survival, that is the necessity of suturing the incision. Thus the surgeon treats the mother as a patient; her death no longer seems to be a precondition for a Caesarean delivery. Again, it is most likely that the scene was drawn according to the reports of surgeons, which the illustrator may have requested. Direct observation is less probable. For one thing, the presence of a male artist at a birth was unacceptable. For another, exact observation would probably have resulted in the representation of the umbilical cord, which is lacking in all the illustrations.[80] The operation itself, on the other hand—the instruments and the incision—corresponds to medical reality.

Not all later illustrators opted for medical realism, however. Our only sixteenth-century illumination of Caesar's birth (fig. 20), was modeled on a Nativity. In fact, it combines two different iconographic traditions of the Nativity. On the right side, it shows the mother, covered by a sheet up to her neck, in bed. This was the earlier schema of the Nativity. The left part of the illumination is taken up by a scene resembling the presentation of Jesus to the three Magi, a somewhat later iconographic development.[81] The combination of the two schemata produces an image of Caesarean birth different from any we have considered so far. Unlike Mary in the various Nativities, the mother here may be dead; the women surrounding the bed seem sad and resigned. But there is no direct evi-

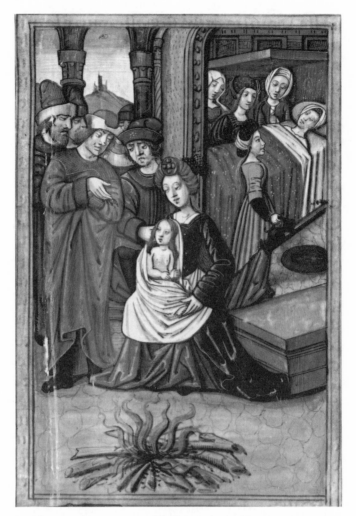

20. The birth of Julius Caesar (Jean Mansel, *Histoires romaines*, Paris, B.N. f. fr. 54, fol. 258r)

dence that a Caesarean birth took place. The long-haired child, wrapped in a sheet, is kept warm in front of a fire. Several men contemplate the child, even point to him.

Men and women are neatly separated in this picture. The women are in the background (except for the female attendant who serves as a support for the child); their attitudes are passive and mournful; in face of death, they can take no action. The men, on the other hand, focus on the new

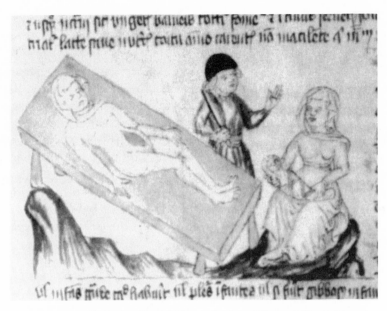

21. A Caesarean birth (London, Wellcome Institute Library, MS 49, fol. 38v)

life, the future ruler. Unlike in most other representations of Caesarean births, in this one there is no feeling of an emergency or even any special activity. The static quality of this picture distances the mother from the birth; she does not receive any medical attention as did the mothers in figures 15 and 16. The child occupies the central position; the mother and the attendants have become marginal.

We are now able to answer the questions asked at the beginning of this chapter. We have seen that the iconography of childbirth (especially of Caesarean birth) produced a tension between iconographic tradition and realistic observation different from that found in the iconography of surgery in general. Illustrations of childbirth were mostly independent of the texts they appeared in but often depended on ancient models. Pictures of Caesarean birth, on the other hand, while also independent of medical texts, developed along different and more diverse lines. Their great diversity is a reflection of a different mode of production. Where illustrators of normal births could rely on an iconographic tradition, those of Caesarean birth had to have recourse to other types of information. Since most of the images are surprisingly accurate from a medical point of view, illustrators must have gathered information from contemporary witnesses, that is, midwives and surgeons. Consequently, the images are more eloquent about medieval life and society than other, more conventional, medical scenes.

As far as gender roles are concerned, we observe an increasing marginality of women in the images. The fourteenth-century midwives, acting so competently and energetically, have no place in the fifteenth century. There is no doubt that male surgeons have taken over the Caesarean operation. Two other illustrations of Caesareans (but not of the birth of Julius Caesar) of the fifteenth and sixteenth centuries confirm this hypothesis: figure 21 shows a male surgeon holding up a surgical knife, and a page from a model book of medical scenes shows a male surgeon performing the actual operation.[82] Women appear only as attendants. The slow incursion of men into obstetrics via the Caesarean operation thus found its own pictorial history.

3 THE MARGINALIZATION OF WOMEN IN OBSTETRICS

The birth chamber was considered the exclusive domain of women, at least up to the eighteenth century.[1] Lyings-in were thus exempt from the male control that extended over almost all other aspects of a woman's life. And yet, as we have seen in the representations of Caesarean birth, for operative deliveries men did enter the birth chamber, and they did so earlier and more consistently than has been recognized in the past. As the evidence shows, midwives were systematically excluded from the Caesarean operation starting about the beginning of the fifteenth century. This exclusion was but the first step in a long series of exclusionary and controlling measures aimed at women in medicine. The marginalization of midwives must be seen in the wider context of misogynistic attitudes in the medieval medical profession and in society at large. The removal of women from positions of relative autonomy to positions under the control of male medical faculties and city administrations becomes especially clear in the fields of obstetrics and gynecology. The independent and competent women practitioners of the earlier Middle Ages are replaced, in the later Middle Ages, by women caught up in a web of medical regulations and municipal ordinances aimed at either prohibiting their practice altogether or at least placing them under total control. Since Caesarean birth was one of the first obstetrical procedures that was lost to female practitioners, the circumstances of this operation can be used as a point of departure for a study of developments in the history of women in medicine. In medicine as well as in historiography the repercussions of many of these developments can still be felt today.

MISOGYNISTIC TRENDS IN THE HISTORIOGRAPHY
OF MEDICINE AND WITCHCRAFT

Medieval misogyny took on so many different forms and was such a constant in the works of male writers that Christine de Pizan, in her *Book of the City of Ladies* (1405), felt compelled to reflect on the discrepancies between the strangely unanimous opinions of male authors and her own observations:

> They [male authorities] all concur in one conclusion: that the behavior of women is inclined to and full of every vice. Thinking deeply about these matters, I began to examine my character and conduct as a natural woman and, similarly I considered other women whose company I frequently kept, princesses, great ladies, women of the middle and lower classes, who had graciously told me of their most private thoughts, hoping that I could judge impartially and in good conscience whether the testimony of so many notable men could be true. To the best of my knowledge, no matter how long I confronted or dissected the problem, I could not see or realize how their claims could be true when compared to the natural behavior and character of women.[2]

Could so many notable men be wrong? Were women not only the instigators of all evil deeds, as the witch-hunters would have it, but also unsuited for responsible positions in society? Or should we say "and *therefore* unsuited for responsible positions in society"? These questions lie at the center of the inquiry into the lives of medieval midwives and female practitioners who were attacked on two fronts at once. On the one hand, they were the victims of the professionalization of medicine, which consisted largely in exclusionary measures directed at women and empiric healers. On the other, midwives and female practitioners were among the prime targets of the witch-hunts. Their knowledge in the areas of contraception and abortion endangered and often cost them their lives.

Much research has been done on the exclusionary practices of the medical profession and the link between the midwife and the witch established by medieval and Renaissance witch-hunters, but scholars have not always recognized exactly how these two areas intersect. The twofold denigration of midwives—by the medical establishment and the witch-hunters—was in fact inspired by a single goal: to discredit and marginalize female midwives and healers.

Understanding of this problem has been hampered by a male scholarly bias in the historiography of medicine as well as in that of witchcraft.

Only recently have some of these problems been brought out into the open.

In 1971, Charles Rosenberg noted that "until comparatively recent times, most medical practice has been in the hands of informal, rural, semi-educated practitioners and such men and women leave few tracks in the archival sand. Thus the history of medical practice has tended to be the chronicle of a self-conscious and comparatively articulate urban elite."[3] Needless to say, this elite was male and paid little attention to the history of women in medicine. Before the work of Mélanie Lipinska in 1900, women made few appearances in the historiography of the medical profession. Since it was this male medical elite (mostly physicians who wrote medical history in their spare time)[4] that was responsible for most of medical historiography, the history of medicine tended to become that of the medical profession, specifically that of the progress in that profession marked by a growing exclusiveness in education and admission to the ranks of licensed physicians. Thus the medieval developments of the medical guilds with their statutes and licensing procedures were hailed as the harbingers of the modern medical profession.[5] The deficiencies of medieval medical practice, which were perpetuated through exclusionary measures (at the expense of often more reasonable "folk" medicine) are rarely seen in connection with—and even more rarely as the result of— the new licensing procedures and statutes that marked the fourteenth and fifteenth centuries. Consequently our knowledge of what empirics, and especially women empirics, actually did is filtered through a screen of prejudices and modern notions of professional medicine.

The historiography of the witch-hunts as well was, until recently, male dominated, although not in the same way as that of the medical profession, which was, in a sense, writing the history of its own "guild." But even well-intentioned historians often lost sight of the fact that in the prosecution of witches the antiempiricist, misogynist, and antisexual obsessions of the church coincided.[6] Thus Gregory Zilboorg sees the profoundly antifeminist *Malleus maleficarum,* a late fifteenth-century handbook for witch-hunters, as "an excellent modern textbook of descriptive clinical psychiatry . . . if the word 'witch' were substituted by the word 'patient' and the devil eliminated."[7] For him, the victims of the witch crazes seem to have been more at fault than the persecutors. If mental illness played a role in the witch-hunts then surely it did so as much on the side of the prosecutors as on that of the prosecuted. As Anne Barstow has shown recently, the idea that women somehow brought the persecutions upon themselves pervades many of the modern accounts of the witch-hunts.[8] Thus Julio Caro Baroja concludes that "a woman usually becomes a witch after the initial failure of her life as a woman," implying that not only did women actually become witches but that they even chose to do so because of some deficiency in their lives, a last recourse for the "unfulfilled woman" as it were.[9] Similarly, Thomas Forbes downplays the perversity of some of the accusations leveled against women when he says, "we have seen how some midwives became involved in witchcraft."[10] Thus caution and an awareness of possible critical prejudices are necessary in approaching the areas in which the demotion of midwives has to be studied.

The Professionalization of Medicine and the Exclusion of Women

That male physicians or surgeons were not allowed in the birth chamber and performed no gynecological exams are two of the received notions in the history of obstetrics and gynecology.[11] They were certainly true for most of the Middle Ages. In the famous trial of the female physician Jacoba Felicie in 1322, the defense counsel argued that "it is better and more seemly that a wise woman learned in the art should visit a sick woman and inquire into the secrets of her nature and her hidden parts, than that a man should do so, for whom it is not lawful to see and seek out the aforesaid parts. . . . A man should ever avoid and flee as much as he can the secrets of women and of her societies."[12]

In the antique and Arabic medical traditions, however, there are clear indications that men assisted in difficult births, that is, they performed embryotomies and possibly even Caesareans and had some functions in gynecology.

In the Hippocratic writings a male physician is mentioned as helping during a protracted birth as well as performing a gynecological exam by inserting a finger into the patient's vagina.[13] The Roman medical writer Celsus (first century A.D.) also specifies that a male physician should perform embryotomies and internal version of the fetus. A male physician also examined women for bladder stones by inserting a finger into the patient's vagina or, if she was a virgin, into the anus.

In Soranus's *Gynecology* the male physician makes several appearances. The description of the causes for difficult labor includes this remark: "or through the inexperience of the midwife or the physician." Somewhat further he says, "In cases of difficult labor the physician should also question the midwife." Finally, he urges that midwives seek the assistance of a male physician for embryotomies.[14] A male presence at difficult births thus seems to be taken for granted.

In the Arabic tradition, several passages in the writings of Abulcasis and Rhazes show men performing or assisting at procedures dealing with difficult births or some gynecological disorders.[15] In a well-known story, Abulcasis mentions an operation for an abdominal tumor that he himself did on a woman. A bizarre aftermath of the operation was the emergence, through the scar, of the bones of several dead fetuses the woman had carried for years.[16]

Rhazes, in a passage in the *Continens* introduced by the term that always identifies his own original remarks, deals with the removal of the secundines by addressing his male reader: "If *you* need to use an iron instrument seat the woman on a chair and let there be a back to the chair." He then specifies that a male practitioner (*mu'ālij*) should use an instrument not unlike the modern speculum to widen the vulva and the cervix.[17] Rhazes also says that he himself performed an extremely painful gynecological operation in which the woman fainted.[18]

Abulcasis, unlike Rhazes, assigns the use of the speculum (of which he provides a sketch) to the midwife.[19] Avicenna in his detailed instructions on the surgical extraction of dead fetuses also only addresses the midwife, although a male advisory function is not excluded.[20] These references, especially for the works of Rhazes, signal a more or less extensive male participation in Arabic obstetrics and gynecology.

But in the medical writings of the medieval Latin West before the late thirteenth century nothing leads to the conclusion that men had functions in obstetrics and gynecology similar to those held by men in the Arabic tradition and in antiquity. Some of the earliest indications that men treated gynecological ailments have been found by Nancy Siraisi in connection with Taddeo Alderotti and his pupils in late-thirteenth-century Bologna. Of Taddeo's one hundred eight-five *consilia*, or descriptions of recommended treatments, ten concern gynecological problems.[21] Guglielmo of Brescia "treated both gynecological problems (if we can judge from the fact that he wrote on breast cancer and tumors of the breast on five separate occasions, and problems of sexual dysfunction)."[22] Writing about a treatment does, of course, not necessarily mean that physicians actually used it, but Siraisi's evidence suggests that they did.

Clearer on the question of the actual performance of an external gynecological exam is John Gaddesden's early-fourteenth-century *Rosa anglica,* which specifies that "ponat medicus vel obstetrix manus comprimendo os stomachi et ventrem" (the doctor or the midwife lays the hand on the stomach or belly to compress it).[23] But the internal gynecological exam was still in the domain of the midwife. It is not until the early fifteenth century that a male physician, Anthonius Guainerius, alludes "to the possibility of a doctor conducting a pelvic examination on a female patient. . . . In the chapter on sterility, he states that if examination is permitted to the physician, he can determine whether sterility is caused by excessive narrowness, width or tortuosity of the mouth of the womb."[24] Caesareans, as we saw in the last two chapters, also started to be performed by men only in the fifteenth century.

Thus a complex picture of men's obstetrical and gynecological activities emerges. It seems that in the later Middle Ages men *regained* some of the functions they had performed in antiquity and the Islamic world, functions they had to wrest away from women who for centuries had been in control of obstetrics and gynecology and thus of their own bodies.

For many women internal gynecological exams evoke—and not necessarily only on a symbolic level—thoughts of the sexual control by men that they experience in their normal lives. In the vulnerable state of illness a woman may thus want to avoid any reminders of male domination. Very often, in fact, men were the cause of the ailments women had to seek help for, as in an extreme example of sexual violence in marriage that can be found in one of the miracles of the Virgin collected by Gautier de Coincy.[25] A husband in Arras, after six months of futile attempts to deflower his young bride, finally, in a fit of rage, takes a knife and mutilates her sexually. When she complains to the bishop he counsels her to remain with her husband, for otherwise, he concludes, she would have no protector. This was, one hopes, an extraordinary case, but it shows nevertheless that a woman could expect little help from men in positions of control. (The woman of Arras is finally saved by the intercession of the Virgin Mary.) No wonder, then, that women had little desire to confide their "secrets," as the counsel of Jacoba Felicie put it, to men. And yet, in the fifteenth century, men make the first inroads into fields closed to them for centuries.

The period of the regaining of male control in certain areas of medicine coincided with efforts to establish medicine as a profession, with all the

exclusionary measures this entailed. But more than a temporal coincidence is involved here, since the professionalization of medicine also led
to a new self-definition of physicians, surgeons, and barbers and to a new
competitiveness regarding areas of permitted activities and fields of competency. Midwives as well as female physicians and surgeons were the
losers in this battle for prerogatives, and their disappearance from images
of Caesarean section marks the beginning of the long struggle on the part
of male doctors and the authorities to banish women from the realm of
medicine.

The professionalization of medicine was closely linked to the rise of the
universities and the establishment of medical faculties. For both Paris and
Montpellier, the earliest references to a medical faculty can be found in
the early thirteenth century, and the first extant medical regulations date
from 1270–74.[26] The granting of medical licenses was a complicated
affair and took place in a biennial ceremony. The charters specified that
no master could present more than two bachelors for the license at any
one time, a proof that only very few students reached this last stage of
their medical education.[27]

The growing exclusiveness of the medical profession led to the frag-
mentation of what had before been a more coherent body of medical
practitioners. The sharpest competition and antagonism existed between
university physicians and surgeons. From 1350 on, doctors required that
all bachelors who hoped to receive a medical license had to take a solemn
oath never to practice manual surgery.[28] Consequently, the surgeons felt
justified in creating their own corporation, the Collège de Saint Côme.
The surgeons of Saint Côme competed for status with the university
physicians. They wore the long robe to set themselves off from the lower
surgeons (*de robe courte*), or the barbers. By 1390, the surgeons were
recognized as "true scholars" by the university, and it seems that at the
beginning of the fifteenth century the surgical corporation gained the
privilege of participating in lectures at the medical faculty of the university.[29] But there was never any real peace between the two groups, for at
the end of the century the university doctors banded together with the
barbers against the surgeons.[30] As a means to woo the barbers, the
learned physicians even allowed the use of the vernacular at autopsies.
The surgeons abandoned some of their functions to the barbers "on the
grounds that such operations would be degrading to surgeons."[31] At the
beginning of the sixteenth century, finally, a semblance of peace was
established between the different professional groups, but it did not last

and the conflicts extended well into the eighteenth century, as Wick-ersheimer pointed out in his introduction to the *Commentaires*.[32]

The turn from the fourteenth to the fifteenth century, then, marked the period of the most intense efforts on the part of the surgeons to gain a status similar to that of the university physicians. Caesarean sections did not belong to the type of operation scorned by surgeons intent on their advancement. This became clear in the illustrations discussed in Chapter 2: all the male surgeons in them wore the long robe of Saint Côme. The efforts to improve the surgeons' status also coincided with the first reports of successful Caesareans.

Oswald Feis discovered in the archives of Frankfurt a document from 1411 that contains a petition to the city council on behalf of a poor old midwife, Mother Guetgin, who was imprisoned for mental illness. The petitioner, a man named Jost von Pern, implores the council to release the midwife. In support of his plea he lists her many accomplishments, the most remarkable being seven Caesarean sections that she had per-formed with "success for mother and child."[33] Given the conditions of abdominal delivery at that period the story sounds unlikely. Neverthe-less, it proves that at least the midwife had a *reputation* of extraordinary skill in this field. It also proves that news of such operations circulated in the early fifteenth century. What better moment, then, for male surgeons to claim a new function for themselves, one that now afforded at least the possibility of gain and prestige?

The first report of a male surgeon having himself performed the opera-tion, that of Piero d'Argellata, postdates the Frankfurt report by only a few years. And it is exactly for that period, of course, that the illumina-tions discussed here faithfully chronicle this transition.

The first official measures restricting the role of women in medicine came from the university faculties, but guilds and corporations did not prove too receptive toward medical women either. Nevertheless, women persisted in trying to find a place for themselves in the many branches of medieval medicine.

Since women were barred from the universities except in Italy, they could not become physicians; but other possibilities were open to them, and they performed a wide variety of healing functions. In medieval French documents many different titles for women in medicine have been recorded: *fisicienne, miresse, chirurgienne, barbière, médecine, guaris-seuse, norrice, sage-femme* (or *ventrière*), and *vieille femme*.[34] *Fisiciennes, miresses,* and *médecines* treated internal ailments, whereas the *chirurgienne,* or surgeoness, was in charge of major operations. The *barbière* could perform minor surgery as well as toothpulling, phlebotomy, and hair-dressing. *Guarisseuse* and *vieille femme* are vaguer terms and probably designate empirics or faith healers. *Sages-femmes,* or *ventrières,* assisted women during childbirth.

For the period between the twelfth and the fifteenth centuries in France, 121 names of women in medicine have been recorded.[35] Of these, about one-third were midwives (including the *aleresses,* or wet nurses) and all of those lived in the fourteenth and fifteenth centuries. *Chirur-giennes* and *barbières* are mentioned in the twelfth century. For the second half of the thirteenth century, fifteen women surgeons and barbers are known by name.[36] It is interesting to note that midwives are mentioned by name only in the later centuries. That is, as long as women were not categorically excluded from other branches of medicine, midwives were not explicitly mentioned. Names were listed only for those women who were surgeons or physicians. But once women were marginalized in the more prestigious medical and surgical professions, actual names of mid-wives start appearing.

In France, the corporations of surgeons did not officially ban women from surgical practice until the edict of Charles VIII in 1484. But, as Danielle Jacquart points out, in most cases women were allowed to take over the office of surgery only if their surgeon husbands had died and the widows did not remarry.[37] In theory, widows of surgeons were legally allowed to practice until 1694.[38] In England, a Guild of Surgeons was formed in 1540, and one of their statutes specified that "no carpenter, smith, weaver, or woman shall practice surgery."[39] Occasionally, women practiced surgery together with their husbands, as did, for example, a certain Guicharde of Lyons whose name is recorded in the year 1267.[40] Several fifteenth-century women successfully assisted their surgeon hus-bands, but when in 1462 the Rheims surgeon Jean Estevenet wanted to enter a monastery and hand over his practice to his wife, the surgical masters of the city took her to court.[41]

One of the statutes of the University of Paris, proclaimed in 1311, addressed itself to both female and male surgeons: "No surgeon or apothecary, man or woman, shall undertake work for which he or she has not been licensed, or approved."[42] But what sorts of skills these surgeons had to have is not quite clear, since documentation on the education of surgeons is very sparse.[43] It is generally believed that the skills subject to approval by a surgical committee were learned by apprenticeship. Surgical treatises are one source of information, of course, but they cover mostly the more complicated functions of a surgeon, and because of their often theoretical nature (especially after the thirteenth century) they probably do not reflect the day-to-day activities of medieval surgeons.

In any case, the surgeoness existed, and we have proof of one of her functions, performing Caesareans, in figures 8, 9, and 10. Women could also perform "minor operative procedures, like cupping."[44] In manuscript Sloane 6, folio 177 (fifteenth century) one can see a woman applying cups (to draw blood) and a cautery.[45] The patient is a man, but in other illustrations in the manuscript the same treatment is applied to female patients.

For women physicians it was very difficult to gain professional approbation. As we saw above, the rise of university medicine made it impossible for women (outside of Italy) to obtain the training necessary for a medical degree. Nevertheless, women practiced medicine in all its forms, including internal medicine, the domain generally reserved for university physicians. Records exist of at least two women who managed to earn the titles of royal physician or surgeon. "Magistra Hersend physica" was one of the physicians of Louis IX and followed him on the crusade in 1249. Her function seems to have been to attend to the queen and other women who accompanied the crusaders.[46] She survived the crusade and was still listed in Parisian records (together with her husband, Jacques, apothecary to the king) in 1259 and 1299. The second case is that of Guillamette de Luys, who appears in a record of 1479 when Louis XI granted her a reward.[47] But women like these were probably the exceptions and too little is known about their education and connections to decide how extensive their functions really were.

More representative of the fate of women healers is the case of Jacoba Felicie. Her trial for unlicensed practice, described in great detail by Pearl Kibre, illustrates how women, at least until they were dragged to court by jealous fellow doctors, could get around official proscriptions. Without explicitly masquerading as a physician, Jacoba gained the confidence of her patients by her competent examinations and diagnoses. She did not demand money until the patient was cured, a practice that probably was unusual for male and female practitioners alike. Several witnesses stated they had turned to Jacoba after a number of licensed physicians had been unable to cure them. But all the support Jacoba received from her patients did no good, and in the final verdict she was found "guilty of willfull disobedience" and, under threat of excommunication and a fine of sixty Parisian pounds, was barred from practicing medicine.[48]

Trials for charlatanism and unlicensed practice continued for the next two centuries, and the defendants were probably not always such capable medical practitioners as Jacoba had been. The medical faculty at Paris gained papal support in their fight for total control over medical practice.[49] As a result of the relentless prosecution of unlicensed healers and of the increasing difficulties for women to obtain a medical education that would then enable them to get licenses, the presence of women in medicine dwindled until Estienne Pasquier could state in the sixteenth century that "one still finds some learned women who, by a special inclination, are drawn to the study of the natural sciences and even of medicine, but very few practitioners."[50]

For midwives, the case was different, of course. General obstetrics did not interest male surgeons until the eighteenth century. Thus midwives continued to assist at births and to perform gynecological exams. What kind of qualifications did they have?

When Soranus answered his question "Who are the best midwives?" he had in mind an ideal type of midwife, probably as rare in antiquity as in the Middle Ages.[51] Here are some of the qualifications he required of a midwife: "A suitable person will be literate with her wits about her, possessed of a good memory, loving work, respectable . . . , sound of limb, and, according to some people, endowed with long slim fingers and short nails at her fingertips. She must be literate in order to be able to comprehend the art through theory too. . . . Now generally speaking we call a midwife faultless if she merely carries out her medical task; whereas we call her the best midwife if she goes further and in addition to her management of cases is well versed in theory." Soranus insisted that the midwife should be competent in all areas of obstetrics and gynecology. He did not think it necessary that a midwife should have had children herself. However, she must be sober and able to keep secrets; she "must not be greedy for money, lest she give an abortive wickedly for payment; she will be free from superstitition." Thus Soranus specified both medical and moral qualifications for his ideal midwife, but the emphasis was clearly on the midwife's medical competence.

Soranus's high medical requirements and especially his insistence on the midwife's literacy no longer fit the midwife's portrait once we enter the Middle Ages. Little is known of the earliest midwives in the medieval

north. The word *heveamme,* which developed into modern German
Hebamme (midwife), is attested in two German poems from the twelfth
and thirteenth centuries that allude to obstetrical examinations performed by these women.[52] In France, the oldest term for a midwife was
ventrière, attested for the first time in 1292.[53] In Italy, the *mulieres Saler-
nitanae* may have been midwives.[54]

Given the low level of female literacy, even toward the end of the
Middle Ages, most midwives must have learned their skills by apprenticeship.[55] There were also many manuals intended for their use. The best
known among these manuals were the works of the Trotula tradition,
which were translated into many languages.[56] But there was also a large
number of anonymous treatises, such as the one analyzed by Pansier in
"Un Manuel d'accouchements du XV°siècle," which concentrated on
fetal positions and how to correct them. More elaborate texts appeared in
the fifteenth and sixteenth centuries, some of them meant for midwives,
such as Roesslin's work, *Der Swangern Frawen,* and some of them addressed to men, such as Anthonius Guainerius's *Tractatus de matricibus.*[57]

But how could midwives profit from these written instructions? In
some cases, groups of literate people may have instructed illiterate practitioners.[58] For late medieval Nuremberg, Merry Wiesner has shown that
the city council assumed that midwives could read;[59] it is therefore not
warranted to conclude categorically that midwives never came into contact with the manuals designed for their instruction.

Another source for the analysis of the midwives' duties and areas of
competency are the canons of various church councils and the regulations
for municipal midwives that appeared in the later Middle Ages. Those
church councils that produced canons dealing with Caesarean sections
placed special emphasis on the midwives' skills and responsibilities. Midwives were forced to make complex decisions on possible surgical delivery and baptism; any misjudgment on their part had serious consequences not only for mother and child but for the midwife's future as
well.[60] Thus the texts of the councils give us one of the earliest testimonies regarding medieval midwives, since they predate any ordinances
and regulations on midwifery by several centuries. On the whole, the
relevant canons seem to place more trust in the midwife's ability than the
later regulations, which are largely of a restrictive nature.

In Germany, regulations of midwifery appeared about a century earlier
than in France. They were characteristic of the large independent towns
with strong municipal governments. Midwives were first mentioned in

Nuremberg in 1381 and "appeared as sworn city officials in the *Amtsbüch-lein,* the list of all occupational groups required to take an annual oath before the council, in 1417."[61] But the first surviving *Hebammenordnung* comes from Regensburg, a town in Bavaria, and dates from 1452.[62] The rationale for the issuing of statutes for midwifery was the "lack and departure" of good midwives and the resulting disorder in the care of women. Candidates for midwifery were examined by a committee of honorable women of the town. To ensure proper care for rich and poor women alike, midwives were required to visit and assist any pregnant woman regardless of her ability to pay. Any delinquent fees would be made up by the honorable townswomen. The only women the midwife was not obliged to care for were Jewish mothers. The *Ordnung* also insisted on sobriety and on patience: no woman, especially if she gives birth for the first time, should be hurried. Forceful dilation, pushing on the stomach to hasten the birth, and urging women too early to help push out the child seem to have been common practice among midwives. As for the Caesarean section, in case the mother dies the midwife is to perform it immediately; no delay or excuse will be accepted. Should both mother and child die, an inquiry will have to show that neglect was not the cause of the disaster. In any case, midwives should use their failure as an opportunity to learn. But if they bury the mother with the child, they will have to pay for this with their lives.[63]

One interesting feature of this ordinance is a reference to unlicensed midwives who try to sneak in at births.[64] They are not condemned out of hand but are permitted at births if in addition a sworn midwife is present.

Another, somewhat later, ordinance from Heilbronn in Swabia requires midwives to call in a physician for difficult births.[65] Midwives are not allowed to perform embryotomies or Caesareans without the presence of a physician; that is, those procedures that involve the use of instruments are now removed from their area of competency.[66] Neither are they allowed to give their patients fragrant waters, balm, or compresses, these remedies being the prerogative of the physician. A late-fifteenth-century addition to the ordinance stated that midwives had to report illegitimate births and abortions to the city government.

The ordinance from Württemberg (1480) discussed in Chapter 1 gives explicit instructions on how to perform a Caesarean and clearly stipulates the possible survival of the mother. In Germany, it seems, where midwives were subjected to official control much earlier than in France, their areas of competency were not limited as severely.

The late fifteenth-century ordinance from Nuremberg, analyzed in detail by Merry Wiesner, fixed the fees for midwives (comparable to those of a skilled craftsman) and forbade married women to enter the profession, probably because they were assumed to be too busy with their own families to do their job adequately. From Wiesner's analysis a picture of the typical midwife emerges: "She was a widow, or an older, unmarried woman, not especially well-off financially as she did not have her own household. The fact that admonitions against married midwives continued indicates that not all were of the marital status considered proper, however."[67]

In none of the early German ordinances do we find any remarks on the training and education of midwives. That they were supposed to learn from older and more experienced colleagues is mentioned in passing, but no specific requirements are enumerated.

Unlike in Germany, in France ordinances regulating midwifery (and thus the "controlled midwife") did not appear until 1560, and this late date may explain the more stringent measures regarding the training and examination of prospective midwives. Richard Petrelli has summarized the course of instruction: midwives with the best reputations were given the title of *matrones jurées* and were in charge of the apprenticeships of future midwives. Paris had four such *matrones*. When the applicant had completed her apprenticeship successfully, the *matrone* issued a *certificat de capacité*. This certificate was then submitted to the king's chief barber-surgeon or his lieutenant and to the priest of the parish. Some theoretical training, offered by the sworn surgeons, was required in addition to the apprenticeship.[68] Thus the midwives were allied with and dependent on the surgical confraternity of Saint Côme, a dependency that in Fasbender's opinion proved extremely harmful for the future of obstetrics.[69] Fasbender does not elaborate on this statement, which is admittedly rather loaded. I believe that he refers to a growing tendency in the male practice of obstetrics of too-frequent surgical interventions and the overuse of instruments. Not for nothing was the man midwife of the eighteenth century referred to as the "Angel of Death."[70] Through our own study we can confirm and clarify Fasbender's uneasy feelings. Male surgeons entered obstetrics via the Caesarean operation; thus the emphasis in the first deliveries performed by men was on a surgical procedure. As a consequence of this early preoccupation with surgical delivery on the part of physicians, surgical intervention became more and more a standardized option in childbirth.[71]

The midwife's chances of getting a medical education consisting of more than observing other midwives at work were very small, and consequently her capacities, especially in the field of surgical delivery, were limited. There seems to be a correlation, however, between the issue of midwifery statutes and the surgical and medical activities allowed to midwives. Thus in France, as we saw in the illustrations, midwives were shown as extremely competent in performing postmortem Caesareans up to about 1400. After that date, when Caesareans on living women seemed at least a possibility, men began to take over. The exclusionary and restrictive measures applied to French midwives are not formalized until much later. They become clearly visible only in the requirements spelled out in the different French ordinances from 1560 to the Revolution, which tended toward questioning and limiting the midwife's autonomy. In almost all of the sixteenth-century ordinances, midwives are required to seek the assistance of a doctor for any birth presenting the slightest difficulty or complication. Regulations fixed in writing thus postdate actual practices by many years. Based on the iconographic evidence, we can conclude that the male takeover of surgical delivery was well under way by the beginning of the fifteenth century.

The late medieval and Renaissance ordinances from France and Germany offered a clear picture of the midwife's official duties and responsibilities. But what of their other, less official but nevertheless well-known functions, such as providing contraceptives and performing abortions and infanticide? It in these areas that midwifery and witchcraft were believed to overlap and it was knowledge in these areas that contributed to the demise of the autonomous midwife.

THE EFFECT OF THE WITCH-HUNTS ON WOMEN IN MEDICINE

Women were the principal targets of the witch-hunters. Of more than a hundred thousand people executed during the witch-hunts, 85 percent were women.[72] One type of woman proved particularly vulnerable to accusations of witchcraft: that of the old "hag," especially if she was a midwife. How did this stereotype of the witch develop? Theological, ideological, and sociological factors all contributed to the creation of a concept of "the witch."

Before 1500, trials for witchcraft occurred in a pattern of peaks and valleys, with the first modest peak sometime between 1315 and 1319 and two more significant peaks about the middle of the fifteenth century and again between 1480 and 1484.[73] The last date marks the issuing of the bull "Summis desiderantes" by Pope Inncocent VIII. In it, he encouraged the two Dominican inquisitors Heinrich Institoris (or Krämer) and Jakob Sprenger to embark on a major witch-hunt. Two years later, the two inquisitors published the infamous *Malleus maleficarum*, which presented the misogynistic and antisexual trends of the witch-hunts in a concentrated form. The *Malleus* repeated and organized material from earlier handbooks and proved extremely influential in the subsequent development of similar texts. These texts reflect the learned tradition of witchcraft and witch-hunting (characterized by an insistence on demonic possession), a tradition which, as Richard Kieckhefer has made clear, must be distinguished from the popular one, which emphasizes evil deeds, or *maleficia*, perpetrated by individuals not necessarily in league with the devil.[74]

A survey of the major works on the witch-hunts shows that theories of witchcraft developed principally in those countries where the learned tradition prevailed and influenced the popular tradition. France and Germany produced a large number of learned treatises on witchcraft, England few. The witch trials themselves also developed differently in these countries. In England, for example, Keith Thomas and Alan Macfarlane have concluded, accusations of witchcraft were very localized, often linked to personal quarrels and revenge.[75] A standard type of accusation involved people who begged at someone's door, were rebuffed, and left muttering curses. If a misfortune, however small, then struck a member of the household, the beggar would be blamed. Thus, as E. William Monter has shown, British scholarship emphasizes the crucial role of *maleficia;* in France, demonological possession came to the fore in showcase trials; in Germany, the emphasis was on panic trials, sometimes of gigantic proportions, which can be traced to the imperial custom of torturing suspects to have them identify their accomplice.[76] The ripple effects of forced denunciations on a large scale, often by children, are easy to imagine.

Generalizations about the European witch-hunts are almost impossible to make. Each region had different characteristics, both in theory and practice. Often witches were burned as scapegoats for specific misfortunes. A plague epidemic in Constance, for example, came to an end only when it was believed that all witchcraft in the region had been destroyed.[77] In other cases, especially the earliest ones in France, many persecutions had political motivations and thus did not single out women.[78] Also, in many regions a strong link existed between heresy and witchcraft, and some scholars believe that the witch-hunts were a natural consequence of the persecution of heretics.[79] Given the large variety in the accusations, the methods of persecution, the types of punishment, the theoretical underpinnings, and the popular beliefs of witchcraft, any uniformity that can be found in all of Europe necessarily takes on special importance. As is well known, the most striking uniform feature of most witch-hunts was their preference for women.

Not all victims of the witch-hunts were women, of course. But Monter has shown that many of the men accused of witchcraft had some connection with suspicious women. He describes the sociological nexus of witchcraft in the Jura region: "Old isolated women; kinship to witches; proximity to witches"—here is the origin of the widening circle of accusations centering on a system that was built on the quick progression in a person's life from a dangerous reputation to accomplice of the devil and his disciples to demonic possession itself.[80] Men were often believed to have been victimized by women and described themselves as having been seduced by witches, as having engaged in witchcraft at the instigation of their wives, for example.

Why were women believed to be more susceptible to witchcraft and why were they the principal victims? The witch-hunts were a means to rid society of threatening elements. Sometimes the threat consisted in the mere existence of a new sociological group. Midelfort shows that demographic changes and a growing tendency to marry later produced such a new group: single women. From 5 percent before the sixteenth century, their percentage in the general population now rose to 15–20 percent. At the same time, widows constituted 10 to 20 percent of the taxpayers.[81] Monter stresses that these women posed a threat to the established order: "If we begin by emphasizing how often these accused witches were elderly widows or spinsters, we can argue that witchcraft accusations can best be understood as projections of patriarchal social fears onto atypical women, those who lived apart from the direct male control of husbands or fathers. These defenseless and very isolated women became the group most often exposed to charges of witchcraft."[82] But the sociological argument is not enough to explain the viciousness of the misogynism evident in the witch-hunts. Other factors were the deep-seated misogynism of the church fathers as well as the idea that women were psychologically and physiologically inferior to men.[83] The writers of the *Malleus* devote many pages to answering the question "Why is it that women are chiefly addicted to evil superstitions?" They do not deny the existence of good women. But they are few and far between (mostly in the Bible). Most women are governed by insatiable lust. Their extreme sexual hunger exposes them to the sexual advances of the devil and makes them his instrument. Only with the help of a demonic pact were women able to perform magic acts, for natural magic was out of their reach: women were considered much too stupid to have any insight into nature.[84] Institoris and Sprenger assemble a large number of misogynistic commonplaces in question 6 of part 1 of their *Malleus maleficarum*. Their special scorn is reserved for midwives, "who surpass all others in wickedness."[85]

This condemnation of midwives brings us to the questions that are most interesting for our present study: Why were midwives and female healers singled out for special persecution? Were all midwives suspected of being witches? Let us first consider the second question.

The *Malleus* did not condemn all midwives out of hand. Let us look at one of its many case histories: "[In Reichshofen] there was a most notorious witch, who could at all times and by a mere touch bewitch women and cause an abortion. Now the wife of a certain nobleman in that place had become pregnant and had engaged a midwife to take care of her, and had been warned by the midwife not to go out of their castle, and above all to be careful not to hold any speech or conversation with this witch."[86] Needless to say, the woman does not take her midwife's advice, leaves the castle, and runs into the witch, who places both hands on the pregnant woman's stomach. As the woman feels the child moving in pain, she returns to the castle where the midwife informs her that it is "already too late." And indeed, when the time for delivery comes, the woman gives birth not to a healthy child but to "separate fragments of its head and feet and hands." This horror was permitted by God to punish the woman's husband, who had not shown enough zeal in the prosecution of witches.

The events in this story are interesting from several points of view. First of all, it is typical for the *Malleus* that a woman should be the scapegoat for her husband's wrongdoing. Second, the punishment is linked to procreation or rather to the prevention of it. Third, the "good" midwife warns of the witch and later blames the disaster at the birth on the evil witch. One gets the impression that "witches" could serve as a kind of malpractice insurance for the good midwife. That is, since mid-wives were in a precarious situation if something went wrong during the birth they may have blamed other women whose reputations were questionable. In any case, this story points to a possible rivalry between midwives, which is also illustrated in another *Malleus* story. A pregnant woman from the vicinity of Strasbourg is approached by a midwife whom she does not trust. She "knew her bad reputation." To placate the untrustworthy midwife the woman falsely promises to request her services for the birth. But when her time comes she calls in a different midwife. A week after the birth the rejected midwife (now called a witch), accompanied by two other women, enters the new mother's room, curses her by touching her abdomen and by "replacing the woman's entrails." As predicted by the "witch," the woman suffers for six months and is then relieved of unclean matters (including brambles, bones, and thorns).[87]

Two important conclusions can be drawn from these stories. First, they aim to portray some sort of professional rivalry between different groups or types of midwives, and second, Institoris and Sprenger claim to believe in the existence of good midwives who could protect women against witches.

How can this conclusion be reconciled with the constant invectives against midwives in the *Malleus*? Clearly, Institoris and Sprenger posited two types of midwives. The good one was in charge of procreation and the protection of pregnant women. The bad one was the enemy of all procreation, for many of the crimes that witches were accused of related to sexual matters or procreation, that is, they made men impotent, incited people to adultery, deprived men of their reproductive organs, and practiced contraception, abortion, and infanticide.

The similarity between the skills of midwives and the supposed magic powers of witches has led to an equation of the midwife and the witch, which, in much of the scholarship on the subject, is made in too facile a manner. After all, the period of the witch-hunts coincides with the period of the first municipal ordinances and regulations for midwives. The city officials and honorable women in charge of formulating and enforcing these regulations did not think that they were dealing with witches. They did exhort midwives, however, not to use superstitious means. The central problem, then, seems to be one of control. The changes made in German midwifery ordinances from the mid-fifteenth to the sixteenth century show that a central concern was to control and to restrict midwives' activities. In addition to the performance of Caesarean section, several other previously accepted activities were now forbidden: dispensing medications, embryotomies of dead fetuses, the use of hooks or other metal instruments, certifying the death of mother and/or child, and finally, diagnosing the diseases through the examination of a patient's blood or urine, that is, all those skills by which surgeons and physicians believed they could distinguish themselves from midwives.[88] As Birkelbach and her colleagues suggest, the regulation that a physician had to be called in at difficult births had no great practical value (since male physicians knew less about childbirth than midwives) but, rather, extended the area of male control over female midwives.

Through these ordinances as well as through accusations of witchcraft, the uncontrolled midwives and practitioners were marginalized, whereas those practitioners who upheld the prevailing antisexual and pro-birth ideology were integrated into the mainstream of society, albeit in inferior—and controlled—positions. It is clear how professionalization and witchcraft intersect: both achieved similar ends with regard to society as a whole and to the healing professions in particular: they marginalized women.

The special skills of midwives and female healers as they related to sexuality and procreation not only were assets used in the service of women's health but also threatened some of the most important values of medieval society: the family and male control over women.[89] Contraception, abortion, and infanticide were some of the means women possessed to control their fertility, the size of their families, and consequently their lives. All of these means were of course condemned by the church, which is not to say, however, that they were not practiced. Let us take a brief look at each of them from a moral-historical perspective.

There are several types of sources for a study of contraception, abortion, and infanticide: religious writings (especially the penitentials), medical writings, and judicial records, such as pardons. All of these sources present their own problems. Medical writings generally belong to a learned tradition and are often far removed from the daily reality of medieval women. Pardons, on the other hand, give us a realistic glimpse of some of the hardships of a woman's life, but they deal, of course, mostly with crimes and thus do not generally include remarks on contraception. The penitentials, used as guidelines for confessors, point up some discrepancies between church theories and practice, since they are often more moderate than the official doctrines of the church and the punishment they mete out is often adapted to real-life situations. From this complex web of sources we will try to unravel those threads which are pertinent to the present study.[90]

Contraception had been practiced since ancient times and no moral judgment was attached to descriptions of the various contraceptive methods in medical texts. In the New Testament (Gal. 5:20), however, Saint Paul condemned the use of *pharmakeia,* or drugs (often magical), and established a link between *pharmakeia* and licentiousness. In Revelation 21:8, fornicators are condemned right after *pharmakoi.* The term *pharmaka,* as John T. Noonan points out, "embraces potions used to affect life or birth." Despite these condemnations, the first three centuries of the Christian era saw few explicit statements on contraception. Influenced by the Stoic idea that all actions must have a well-defined purpose, the church posited that sexual intercourse can be justified only if it has a procreative purpose. In the fourth century, Saint Jerome described contraception as homicide ("Others, indeed, will drink sterility and will murder a man not yet born"), and Augustine listed offspring (*proles*) as one of the three goods of marriage. In Augustine's hierarchy of values, however, procreation comes only after fidelity and continence: having children spiritually is more valuable than having real children.[91] Augustine vehemently condemned "poisons of sterility" as destructive to the goods of marriage in a passage that was known throughout the Middle Ages as the *Aliquando.*[92] Jerome's definition of contraception as homicide became the prevalent one, possibly because he used the expression *drinking* sterility, and most contraceptives were indeed potions. Another important milestone in the condemnation of contraception was a tenth-century text (*Si aliquis*) by Regino of Prüm, which helped anchor the equation of contraception and homicide in canon law, an equation, however, that many considered excessive and that was not universally and at all times accepted.[93] Nevertheless, in many penitentials contraception was referred to as *maleficia,* a term that also had connotations of pagan magic. Not only were the women who desired contraceptives condemned there: those aiding her in procuring them were just as guilty.

From ancient times certain types of *maleficia* had been linked to women. Women were accused of achieving their evil designs by poison, by the throwing of lots, by incantation, by the production and destruction of waxen images, and the like. Rendering men impotent was believed to be one of the specialties of the pagan and medieval *striga,* or witch. Personal jealousy and a desire for vengeance after being left by a lover supposedly moved two women in late-fourteenth-century Paris to cause male impotence by various ointments and waxen images.[94] While the devil can physically remove the male member,[95] witches habitually cast a "glamor" over it so that the men believe their penis has vanished. This technique is illustrated in the story of a young man of Regensburg who lost his member after breaking up with his girlfriend. When he consults a woman in a tavern about his problem she suggests that his girlfriend is a witch who has made his penis disappear. The young man returns to his girlfriend demanding the restitution of his member. The girl, naturally, claims total ignorance in this matter and "relents" only when the man is about to strangle her. She is thus persuaded to touch him between the thighs, saying, "Now you have what you desire." Immediately afterward the young man feels that his member has reappeared.[96] One can see how the fear of impotence, a specifically male fear, would lead to belief in such a story. To have control over sexual performance meant also to have control over procreation. While impotence and sterility were feared by men as limiting their power, contraception could be seen by women as increasing their power.[97] Based on such stories as the ones just cited the different meanings of *maleficium* fused semantically and, in the title of that most pernicious text of the witch-hunts, *Malleus maleficarum,* were clearly assigned to the female sex.

Women were in charge of most contraceptive means, but a distinction has to be made between sexual practices that may have a contraceptive effect (for example, oral or anal sex) and means that are designed only for contraception.[98] In the early penitentials (up to 813), there are, according to Pierre Payer, no explicit condemnations of either contraceptive sexual practices or potions. But, of course, enough later canons existed that condemned any form of contraception. From L. Flandrin's study, "Contraception, mariage, et relations amoureuses," it becomes clear that "unnatural acts", that is, those sexual practices that precluded procreation, were extremely widespread and vehemently censored by the church.

A variety of contraceptive means were available to medieval couples. The ancient and the Arabic medical traditions recommended talismans as well as various herbal spermicides, pessaries or suppositories (soaked, for example, in mint juice), and potions. Jumping backward (nine times) after intercourse may expel the seed. Fumigation with the smoke of a burning mule's hoof is also recommended.[99] Most of the contraceptives are meant for women, but a few were meant for men, such as oiling the penis with cedar oil.

What is interesting in the transmission of contraceptive knowledge is the separation between the teachings of the church and the medical texts of the time. A striking example is Albertus Magnus, who gives no explicit recipes for contraceptives (although he mentions coriander, rue, and lettuce as anaphrodisiacs), but in his explanations of sterility becomes a fertile source for contraceptive knowledge (*malgré lui,* perhaps?).[100] In any case, he keeps his moral judgments neatly separated from his medical teachings.[101]

Thus medieval attitudes toward contraception were ambiguous. Condemned unequivocally in the writings of the church, contraceptive means were transmitted in medical writings and in the popular tradition. According to Noonan, contraception was not a major social problem, since it was hardly mentioned in secular law. The major heresy that could have posed a threat to the perpetuation of the species, the Cathars, had been eradicated by 1260. "There were economic reasons for individuals to limit births. But plague, famine, and war affected western Europe often enough in this period so that there was no serious population pressure. It [contraception] was practiced chiefly to avoid impoverishment."[102] Nevertheless, contraception continued to be proscribed, and it was not until the eighteenth century that the equation of contraception and homicide was banned from theological writings.[103]

These conclusions have by no means been universally accepted. The militant German scholars Heinsohn and Steiger try to refute Noonan's claim of the social unimportance of contraception. It was the possibility of depopulation, brought about by the fourteenth-century Great Plague, they claim, that turned contraception into a major threat to the ruling classes. The witch-hunts were predicated on the desire to assure the production of people.[104] The proof that the authors provide for a carefully planned campaign for an increase of the labor force are minimal. Nevertheless, as I mentioned earlier, many of the accusations leveled against witches centered on the skills and functions of midwives.

Women who were accused as witches often lived on the margins of society. Married women were not persecuted as often as unmarried women. Now, one of the developments of the fifteenth century was a new theory, elaborated by Martin Le Maistre (1432–81), on marital intercourse that posited that "not every copulation of spouses not performed to generate off-spring is an act opposed to conjugal chastity."[105] Even though Le Maistre's views were slow to take hold, they eventually gained general acceptance. In practice this meant that a childless marriage was not immediately suspect. But the slightly looser interpretation of the condemnation of contraceptive means did not extend to extramarital intercourse and pregnancy. Again, we encounter the problem of control. The example cited earlier of controlled midwives versus uncontrolled midwives can now be supplemented by the opposition between controlled and uncontrolled intercourse. Witches were clearly associated with the latter and thus posed an extraordinary threat to established marriage. Sex outside of marriage must be punished, and any form of birth control would make it possible to remove the most certain proof of sinful conduct: children. Thus the production of children was not a value at all; the invective of Institoris and Sprenger was directed against those women capable of hiding, or helping other women hide, the consequences of their insatiable lust.

One of the main tenets of the *Malleus* was women's sexual insatiability and their consequent susceptibility to diabolical influences, specifically their desire to copulate with the devil. Hansen places Institoris and Sprenger's insistence on the sexual nature of diabolical possession in the context of ascetic and misogynistic currents of the later Middle Ages.[106] If witches had (sterile) intercourse with the devil they naturally posed a threat to the goods of marriage. But again it seems that the campaigns against midwives who were believed to be witches were set in motion not primarily by a desire for the increase of population but rather because exaggerated, even morbid, views of sex led to the violent prosecution of those knowledgeable of contraceptive means. A consideration of one of the other supposed crimes of witches, infanticide, will clarify this position.

Pope Innocent's bull *Summis desiderantes* insisted that witches "cause to perish the off-spring of women."[107] This indictment could refer to either abortion or infanticide. Two years later, Institoris and Sprenger specified the midwives' supposed crimes in part I, question II of the *Malleus:* "That witches who are midwives in various ways kill the child conceived in the womb, and procure an abortion; or if they do not this offer new-born children to devils. Here is set forth the truth concerning four horrible crimes which devils commit against infants, both in the mother's womb and afterwards. And since the devils do these things through the medium of women, and not men, this form of homicide is associated rather with women than with men." Interestingly, the authors go on to describe natural means of contraception, such as certain herbs, which do not belong to the province of witches. Unnatural acts, including abortion, miscarriage, and the devouring of children, are ascribed to the midwife-witches. Institoris and Sprenger conclude, "No one does more harm to the Catholic Faith than midwives."[108] And at the height of the witch-hunts, one of the preeminent inquisitors, Henri Boguet, posed a question similar to that found in the *Malleus:* "How do midwives, if they are witches, kill the children they deliver?"[109] At a trial in Briançon in 1437 the precise description of an infant's murder in his cradle would provide an answer to Boguet's question. The child was killed; his body was then mixed with "nightly pollutions," menstrual blood, and pubic hair and used for ritual purposes.[110] This last point is crucial, for it distinguishes infanticide by witches from that committed by other women.

Evidence for the practice of infanticide exists for many different regions and centuries, but most of it involves cases of mothers who killed their own infants. Forced by social and economic pressures, many women apparently saw no other solution. Emily Coleman, in "Infanticide in the Early Middle Ages," based on the ninth-century polyptych of Saint Germain-des-Près, has shown that infanticide was practiced as a means of population control. The victims were mostly female. This also holds true for fifteenth-century Florence, where the proportion of surviving girls was abnormally low.[111] In every respect, infanticide was a female crime. The principal offender was the unwed mother. Since midwives were obliged by law to report any illegitimate births, their help was not sought by unmarried pregnant women. Efforts to conceal pregnancies and to dispose of the evidence—the babies—led to horrifying crimes of despair. In "L'infanticide à la fin du moyen âge," Brissaud lists a large number of cases of infanticide, many of them heartbreaking examples of the isolation and helplessness of lower-class women. Some women baptized their infants before killing them, a practice that would reduce their punishment if they were found out but that also may have helped assuage their mental anguish. The discovery of a dead baby usually led to extensive searches for the guilty woman; these searches involved the intimate examination of suspected women and bore some resemblance to the witch-hunters' search for the witches' mark, a degrading and sexually charged procedure.[112]

Since the time of Charlemagne infanticide had been treated as homicide. Under the reign of Saint Louis a first offense of involuntary infanticide, such as accidentally suffocating a child in bed with its parents, was punished by prison, but a repeat offender would be punished by death: she would be burned or buried alive.[113] From the pardons issued to women guilty of infanticide one gets a slightly less grim picture. If a woman was too young to know what she was doing, if the child died accidentally or was born dead, if penances were already imposed (such as a pilgrimage to Rome), if she had children who needed her or if she promised to marry the father of the child—in all these cases clemency might be expected.[114]

There are important differences between the cases of infanticide just discussed and the often fantastic accounts of infanticide supposedly committed by witches. The fact that poverty was one of the most frequently cited extenuating circumstances in the penitentials seems to indicate that mothers could expect at least some sympathy if their motives were economic. On the other hand, a prostitute who wanted to hide her "perversity" by killing her child had no hope for leniency.[115] Similarly, for witches, no extenuating circumstances could be cited, but here because of the belief that their killing of children involved sexually perverse rituals. The ingredients listed in the above-mentioned trial at Briançon give us some idea of how the witch-hunters imagined these rituals. The witches' brew was a sexual brew and led, in the inquisitors' imagination, to orgies of copulation with the devil.

Midwives, then, are condemned because they are women and as such ready to submit sexually to the devil; but they also possess the sexual expertise that allows them to control men and other women. They assume control not only over their own reproductive functions but also over those of their victims. And it is exactly this control that municipal ordinances on midwifery are designed to wrest away from women. As Merry Wiesner has shown, "midwives appear most often in the city council records (*Ratsbücher*) in connection with criminal cases, particularly abortion and infanticide," which they were obliged to report.[116] Midwives were thus employed to spy on and denounce the unfortunate women who had to bear the shame of an illegitimate pregnancy.

Midelfort points out that midwives formed one group of the population that was most often denounced by tortured suspects.[117] He does not attempt, however, to give any reasons for the notoriously bad reputation of midwives. The principal reason that midwives were feared and denounced was clearly their knowledge, or at least their claims to knowledge, of means and techniques relating to sexual performance, procreation, and the prevention of procreation. But another reason for the popular dislike of midwives may have been their official function as spies in sexual matters for the authorities. Thus the midwives were caught between conflicting obligations. On the one hand, their task was to help and protect women and their offspring; but on the other hand, they had to betray and expose to severe punishment the weakest members of the group entrusted to their care. This supposed position of power contributed to the midwives' downfall.

No other campaign in history was so clearly directed against women as the witch-hunts. Especially for women in medicine the long-term effects of the witch-hunts were disastrous. Given the state of medieval medicine, diagnosis and therapy were tentative at best, and it was easy to ascribe medical failures to the evil charms of witches. Women could be removed from positions of control and power without much ado, and most women were probably wary of assuming such positions even if they had the chance to do so. It is hardly surprising therefore to find "few female medical practitioners" in the sixteenth century, as Estienne Pasquier remarked.[118]

SPECIAL PROBLEMS OF CAESAREAN BIRTH

As early as the fourteenth century, before the theoretical crystallization of the image of the witch, women were accused of stealing stillborn babies or of killing newborns by their touch.[119] In cases of Caesarean birth, the conditions for these supposed crimes must have been considered ideal. The mother would most likely be already dead when the child was delivered; the family might be in such distress that they would not pay attention to what happened to the baby. But, most important, the decision of whether to perform a Caesarean at all would be up to the midwife. Thus the midwife had more power in the extraordinary circumstances of Caesarean birth than in those of normal childbirth, where her position would be at best that of an auxiliary.

One of the most frequently cited accusations against midwives was that the newborn had died unbaptized. The same accusation was leveled against supposed witches. In the 1437 trial at Briançon, one of the principal points of the prosecution was that the child was *sine baptismo defunct[us]*.[120] In 1587, a midwife confessed to a whole series of crimes against unborn and newborn children. In every case, the midwife spec-

ified, the devil forced her to kill the children before they were baptized.[121] These crimes were considered especially heinous because it was
the medieval midwife's responsibility to see to it that the newborn was
baptized.[122] The city of Nuremberg even composed a special baptism
ordinance that was distributed to midwives.[123]

Now, we recall that those canons of various church councils that dealt
with Caesarean birth laid a special stress on the midwife's obligation to
perform baptism. The situations in which a Caesarean was indicated were
clearly the most critical ones, resulting as they did in the death of the
mother and frequently of the child. More than in normal births, then,
mothers and children involved in Caesarean births were at the mercy of
the midwife. Not only the possible physical salvation of the child but its
spiritual salvation as well lay in her hands alone. It now becomes clearer
why male surgeons replaced female midwives in Caesarean birth earlier
than in normal childbirth. One of the motivations that prompted the
male takeover was the distrust of midwives. Would they perform their
duties as to the baptism of the newborn? The answers to this question
ranged from doubtful to negative, since as early as the second half of the
fourteenth century executions for the killing of unbaptized infants are
reported.[124]

In addition to the supposed worry about the spiritual welfare of
mother and child, professional rivalries and the efforts on the part of
established male physicians and surgeons to control female medical practitioners played the largest roles in the marginalization of women. Theological and medical-professional reasoning go hand in hand for the
problems associated with Caesarean birth. An examination of two midwives' ordinances from 1452 and 1552 (printed in 1555) confirms these
points.[125] As outlined above, the changes show a systematic restriction of
the midwives' activities. The Caesarean section plays a central role here.
The 1452 ordinance specifies that the midwife, should she feel in need of
help for a Caesarean, should call in an especially qualified *woman*. The
motivation for the composition of the ordinance (the "disorder" [*unor-
dnung*]) may imply that midwives hesitated in the performance of a
Caesarean: believing the mother to be still alive they apparently refused
to perform a Caesarean in time for the child to be baptized. Thus
Caesarean section is one of the most sensitive issues in this context.
Accordingly, the sixteenth-century ordinance specifies that a *doctor der
artzney,* that is, a male physician, must be called in for a Caesarean. He is

now in charge of Caesareans and any other deliveries involving the use of surgical instruments, which midwives are no longer allowed to use.[126]

Together with the fact that the control of midwives was now in the hands of the city council (as opposed to the "honorable women" of the first ordinance) this male takeover of Caesarean sections marked a decisive step in the marginalization of midwives.

Caesarean birth is useful as a touchstone for an investigation into the marginalization of women in medicine because the developments described in this chapter can be observed first in the context of that operation and in the images depicting it. For centuries, male obstetrical intervention was characterized by the use of instruments, which became a symbol of the supposed male superiority in terminating a difficult birth.[127] It was in the context of Caesarean sections that the male prerogative regarding the use of instruments was spelled out explicitly for the first time.

In a period when the consequences of the Great Plague led to tightening requirements in the medical profession and, at the same time, to a search for scapegoats in society, women had to relinquish their places of relative autonomy and authority in the healing professions.[128] The same two currents that have been studied separately as consequences of the fourteenth-century plague combined forces and resulted in the demotion of medical women. The professionalization of medicine and the witchhunts worked together to ensure male control over women in medicine.[129] Through the marginalization of midwives and their knowledge of contraception, men claimed control over women's reproductive functions, a control they have been slow to relinquish. Thus, in the fourteenth century, the seeds were planted for ideas and attitudes that still affect women today.

4 SAINTLY AND SATANIC OBSTETRICIANS

In a special cult in seventeenth-century Swabia, Saint Roch, the fourteenth-century saint generally in charge of plague victims, came to function as a "celestial gynecologist."[1] This new competency assigned to him was due to an iconographic confusion that, by analogy, interpreted Saint Roch's plague wound (usually located on his upper thigh) as the female genitalia.[2] To many childless and suffering women the shape of the wound apparently recalled their own organs, which were the cause of their distress. The development of the special cult of Saint Roch as gynecologist thus centered on the idea of a wound or opening, which also appeared on votive offerings in chapels dedicated to Saint Roch: these were metal toads with baby faces and large vulvalike openings on their backs believed to be substitutes for representations of the uterus.[3] The imagery of this cult thus was sexually charged. Saint Roch's gesture could also suggest that he was pointing to his own genitals: consequently, the worshipers who adopted this cult saw male and female sexuality represented in the same figure. In an additional twist to this complicated pattern, the next step in the development of this cult consisted in the association of the toad with the viper or dragon of Saint Margaret, the special patron saint of childbearing women. The sexual significance of the dragon in the story of her martyrdom is obvious: he represented the enemy of her chastity, and he was split open through her prayers. It appears that an analogy between the dragon's and the toads' wounds was established in the popular imagination.[4] As a result, chastity and sexuality could be represented simultaneously in one and the same votive offering.

From this example, illustrating the working of the popular religious imagination, two points emerge that are important to the study of Caesarean birth and that will structure this chapter: the roles of some saints and the Virgin as obstetricians and the creation of rather bizarre analogies that may have led to the depiction of the Antichrist's birth as a Caesarean.

"APERTURA MIRABILIS":
MIRACULOUS CAESAREANS

If in the official writings of the church pregnant women found few sympathetic supporters, miracle collections offered more comfort. In addition to the Virgin, some saints, for example Saint Margaret or Saint Hyacinth, were special patrons of childbirth. Others helped in childbirth only occasionally.[5] In both categories we find a few miracles in which mothers survived a Caesarean delivery (usually of a dead fetus).

The Virgin was in charge of aiding women in all sorts of misfortunes surrounding childbirth. In one case, a woman lost her child accidentally after the death of her husband; now unprotected, she was accused of having performed an abortion. After being thrown by her accusers from a bridge she was rescued from the torrents by Notre Dame de Rocamadour.[6] This miracle not only illustrates the powers of the Virgin but paints a rather dark picture of a pregnant woman's fate without the protection of her husband. In the case of an accident to the fetus she is left at the mercy of her husband's family who, in this particular story, only debate the ways to get rid of her (fire or water?), not the question of her guilt or innocence.

The Virgin of Rocamadour was a preferred patroness of childbirth. In one of her miracles a woman is delivered by a Caesarean. In order to give the flavor of this type of miracle I will translate it in its entirety:

> Of a woman who suffered every day the pangs of childbirth. I cannot omit an astonishing and curious miracle of a kind that one has never heard of before. A woman of the country of the Goths had been pregnant for almost thirty months; every day she was tormented by the pangs of childbirth but could not give birth. Her parents, of whom she was the only child, belonged to the confraternity of Notre-Dame de Rocamadour. Their sorrow was immense, they could not stop crying; it was as if their daughter were already dead. Those who heard tell of such a new and awful sickness were astonished; those who saw the sick woman were filled with pity. This

terrible act by God induced fear in all those who saw it because it seemed that He had forgotten his own pity and the woman's weakness. In this poor woman the words were fulfilled "in pain you shall bring forth children." But she would have been only too happy to give birth even though childbirth is painful, and she would have been happy, considering that pain [i.e., of giving birth] as nothing. Therefore she ardently desired to die, even though death is full of bitterness and she proclaimed those who could die happy. For she was dying alive and considered death sweeter than her pain because death lasts only a moment. At the moment of giving birth every woman is, in a sense, at death's door; what pain, then, must this woman have felt who suffered continually the pangs of childbirth? Clearly, this was the greatest pain ever endured by any woman. Her parents tried to move to compassion the merciful Mother of God, knowing well that fervent and constant prayer penetrates the heavens and pacifies the supreme Judge. Since the illness was extraordinary it could only be cured in an extraordinary manner by the faithful physician. Miraculously the stomach of the poor woman opened, contrary to nature and without the help of a doctor. The dead and already putrid child was extracted in pieces and the mother was completely healed. She came to the church of Rocamadour to give thanks to her benefactress. And since she belonged to that uncouth nation that does not know any shame she gladly showed her still open wound. She did not stop singing the praise of the powerful Virgin.[7]

The last detail, that of showing the wound, is extremely important in the context of childbirth miracles. This type of miracle was problematic from several points of view. First, if the birth was the answer to a prayer for fertility, it was difficult to link it directly to a saint's shrine, since it took place nine months later and often at quite a distance from the shrine.[8] Second, usually no visible mark remained that could be shown in thanksgiving to the saint or Virgin. An abdominal delivery thus plays a special role. Even though the showing of the wound or scar may be considered immodest, it nevertheless fulfills the all-important function of giving visible proof of a miracle.[9]

If in the miracle of Rocamadour the woman shows off her still-open wound, the heroine of a miracle of Saint Vulframmus can show more restraint: her wound is just sufficiently healed to be decent, but, the hagiographer specifies, "the sign of the division remained so that God's virtue and that of his servant [Saint Vulframmus] would forever be manifest."[10] Nothing in Saint Vulframmus's life especially qualified him for aiding pregnant women. The most notable deed of this eight-century bishop had been the conversion of Frisia. The list of his miracles includes the usual collection of children revived after drowning, sailors rescued in a storm at sea, and soldiers protected during battle. And yet, in this one case, his saintly intervention leads to an obstetrical procedure described in unusual detail; in that, this miracle differs dramatically from the more general and conventional descriptions used for the saint's other miracles. Here is the most dramatic moment: "After insistent prayers [to Saint Vulframmus] her belly was swelling up from the pectoral bone to the navel when—wonderful to tell—it divided itself across the middle like a field newly plowed. Her cries made people flock around and look at her without modesty. After some consultation they opened her belly further and pulled the flesh and bones of the putrid child out of the half-dead woman's body. When this was done, the woman again prayed to the saintly patron who had delivered and completely healed her."[11] Her scar, the visible sign of her salvation, remains and she shows it to anyone who wants to see it. From this miracle it becomes clear that a Caesarean was considered the last resort for a woman suspected of being pregnant with a dead fetus. Even though the location of the incision does not seem to be accurate, the details suggest some familiarity, on the hagiographer's part, with such procedures.

A similar miraculous deed (*gesta miracula*), this time performed by a church father who was also a *medicus,* Paul of Merida in Lusitania, is recorded for the seventh century. At the time when Paul is bishop of Merida the wife of one of the noblemen of the city falls sick: her child has died in her womb. After having lost all confidence in physicians, the husband approaches Paul. Interestingly, the husband first approaches him because Paul is a holy man, not because he is a physician. Paul first refuses to heal her with his own hands lest "wicked men will throw this matter up to me." He finally relents, prays a whole day at the church of the virgin Saint Eulalia, and then "laid his hands on the sick woman in the name of the Lord, and, trusting in God, very carefully made a very small incision with a sharp scalpel and withdrew in sections, member by member, the already corrupt body of the infant. The woman, already almost dead and only half-alive, he at once restored safely to her husband with the help of God and bade her henceforth not to know her husband: for at whatever time she should know the embraces of her husband worse perils would come upon her. Nevertheless they fell at his feet and thanked him and promised to observe in detail everything the man of God had commanded." Prayers and immense joy follow this miraculous deliverance.[12]

This incident is one of the extremely rare detailed accounts of a Caesarean for late antiquity. What is remarkable here is that the woman's body is not opened miraculously but rather that divine support is given to a medical procedure that is executed by a bishop-physician. By repeating the word *subtilis* (subtle or careful) the author insists on the extreme skill necessary for such an operation: "mira subtilitate incisionem subtilissmam subtili cum ferramento fecit."[13] Paul also gives advice to the couple that is clearly in the interest of the woman. Although newly married, she does not have to pay the "marital debt" at the risk of a future pregnancy that could endanger her life. This story highlights not only the miraculous powers of a holy physician but also shows great comprehension of women's risks and problems by integrating the perils of intercourse and pregnancy into a compassionate and nonmisogynistic context.

The degree of direct saintly participation varies in all these stories. On the whole, there is a progression from divinely guided medical intervention to pure miracle. While Paul of Merida performed the Caesarean himself, albeit with the help of God, Saint Vulframmus intervenes only partially, that is, he opens up the woman's abdomen only to indicate what kind of procedure is needed; the operation of removing the fetus is performed by humans. But in the most recent story, that of Notre-Dame of Rocamadour, the Virgin seems to do most of the "work" and any human help is hidden under some vague passive constructions (*puer . . . extractus est,* "the boy was extracted").

Another miracle story (and especially its transformation) gives us further insight into the conditions of medieval marriage and pregnancy. It is a story of love, jealousy, and suicide. A husband teases his pregnant wife by claiming to have a mistress much more beautiful than she. "If this is true," his wife retorts, "I will pierce myself with this knife." The husband, whose sense of humor is questionable, insists that it is so. Without hesitation the wife plunges the knife into her uterus in order to kill herself and the child. Suddenly the husband realizes what is happening; he starts beating his chest and tearing his hair: he now knows that he has lost not only his wife but also his child. In vain he tries to extract the knife and prays ardently to the Virgin. As his wife's body is perforated by the knife, so, he states in his prayer, his own body is now perforated by pain. Without delay the Virgin answers his prayer and the husband now can extract the knife which had pierced the woman's spine. Everyone weeps and the woman is saved. The husband whose callousness caused the entire disaster is seen as a repentant sinner; the wife is, all along, a victim (if a strong-minded one).[14]

A fourteenth-century transformation of this twelfth-century story gives quite different roles to both husband and wife. Here, the husband is so devoted to the Virgin that he secretly builds an altar for her at which he prays at night when he thinks his wife is asleep. The wife, who is pregnant, wakes up one night to an empty bed. The next morning she complains to him by saying, "Am I not beautiful enough for you? Why do you love someone else?" The husband's answer, that he indeed loves someone far more beautiful than his wife (he secretly meant the Virgin, the author adds), enrages the wife even more. The rest of the story resembles the earlier version except for one important detail: the child, after it is born, forever carries the sign of the wound inflicted by his mother on his forehead.

The later story transforms the wife into a suspicious shrew and the husband almost into an saint. The imaginary mistress of the first story has become the "real" mistress, the Virgin.[15] The mother's guilt and the Virgin's miraculous intercession are forever inscribed on the child's forehead. Thus the wife has been doubly defeated by the Virgin.

The knife, which, in the story of Paul of Merida, had been the instrument of salvation, becomes here the instrument of sin and mutilation. In one of the miracles in the collection of Gautier de Coincy, a woman from Arras is sexually mutilated with a knife by her husband because he is unable to deflower her. The sexual symbolism of the knife is only too obvious here. In medieval iconography, the knife is especially prominent in images of the circumcision and of course in those of Caesarean birth. In the pictures of Caesarean birth studied in Chapter 2, the knife was always central and its size was sometimes so exaggerated that it looked like an enormous sword. The contamination of these two patterns, that of mutilation and destruction and that of Caesarean birth, is in my opinion at least partially responsible for the creation of one of the most striking and disturbing images in late medieval iconography: the birth of the Antichrist by Caesarean section. Here the idea of the unnaturalness of Caesarean birth finds its most graphic expression.

THE BIRTH OF THE ANTICHRIST

Images of the Antichrist's birth by Caesarean first appeared in German woodcuts in the second half of the fifteenth century. These woodcuts were used in a rather restricted area: roughly in the triangle formed by Augsburg, Nuremberg, and Strasbourg. One of the woodcuts (fig. 24) made its way to Spain. Figures 22–27 show all the major versions found

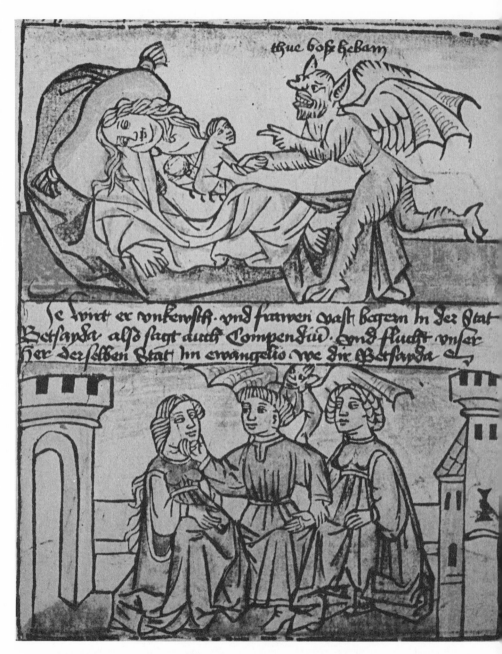

22. The birth of the Antichrist (*Endkrist*, Collection Otto Schäfer, fol. 2v)

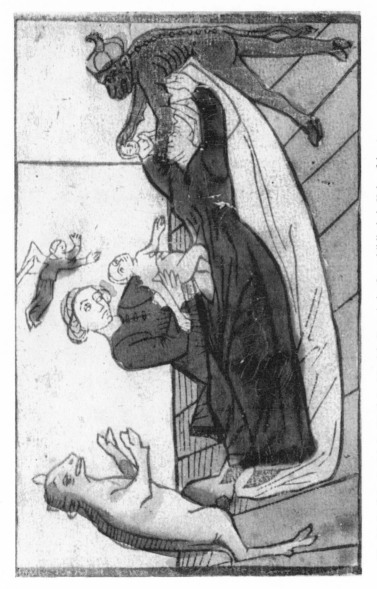

23. The birth of the Antichrist (*Entkrist*, Munich, Bayerische Staatsbibliothek, Xyl. 1, fol. 2r)

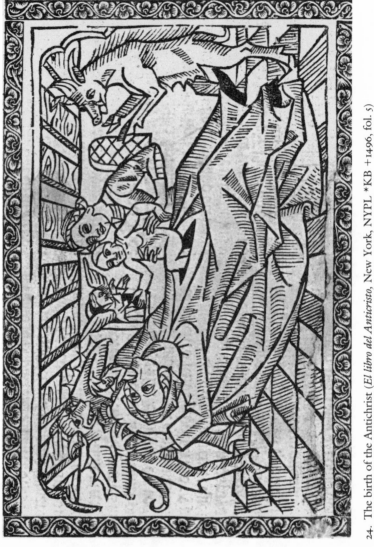

24. The birth of the Antichrist (*El libro del Anticristo*, New York, NYPL *KB +1496, fol. 5)

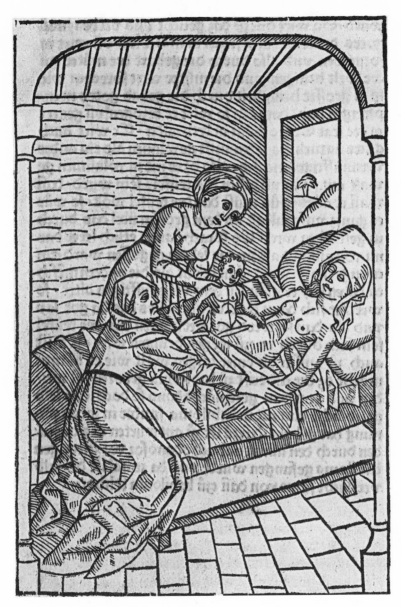

25. The birth of the Antichrist (*Seelenwurzgarten*, New York, Pierpont Morgan Library, PML 199 Ch L f 490, fol. dd6v)

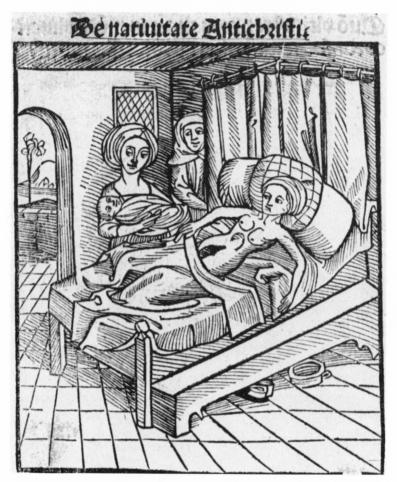

26. The birth of the Antichrist (Pseudo-Methodius, *Opusculum divinarum revelationum*, New York, NYPL, Stuart *KB 1504)

in block books as well as in printed books. Even though these images are part of a purely iconographic tradition, only a combined study of both the textual *and* the iconographic traditions of the Antichrist's birth will provide a clue to these rather bizarre images in which devils function as midwives and mothers are depicted with gaping wounds in their stomachs.[16] The body of primary and secondary works dealing with the Antichrist is immense;[17] I will therefore concentrate on those textual elements that emphasize the context and manner of the Antichrist's conception and birth.

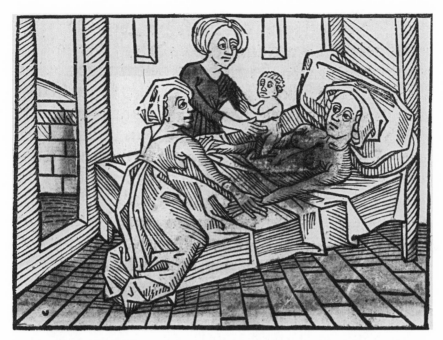

27. The birth of the Antichrist (*Seelenwurzgarten*, San Marino, Huntington Library, RB 101792)

From the beginning, the Antichrist's life was defined both as analogous and opposite to Christ's: he would imitate Christ in a perverted manner. Before the creation of a coherent legend of the Antichrist's life, or a vita, some details about the Antichrist's birth appeared in a commentary on the Apocalypse (first century A.D.) where his emergence was equated with the rising of the beast out of the abyss described in Rev. 11:7.[18] Early on, the Antichrist was also linked to the tribe of Dan as it appears in Jacob's benediction and prophecy: "Dan shall be a serpent in the way, a viper in the path, that bites the horse's heels so that the rider falls backward" (Gen. 49:17). This image captured the medieval imagination; it appears in countless passages of the church fathers as well as in vernacular texts. In the third century the exegetes Irenaeus and Hippolytus provided a first codification of some important traits of the Antichrist's life: the Antichrist is Satan's son; in every detail he is the opposite of Christ and the church.[19] This last idea opened the door to a variety of historical interpretations: the Antichrist is a Jew, a heretic, or, later on, a Moslem.[20] But it also gave the impetus for the creation of a vita for the

Antichrist that would resemble in its structure the traditional saint's life that in turn was modeled on the Life of Christ. The late-seventh-century Syrian writer known as Pseudo-Methodius was the first to use at least some elements of a vita. He specified that the Antichrist would be born in Chorozaim, would be raised in Capernaum, and would reign in Bethsaida.[21] He also used the image of the Antichrist as the viper of the tribe of Dan. Pseudo-Methodius's text, together with other exegetical and popular traditions, strongly influenced one of the most important works on the Antichrist: the *Libellus de ortu et de tempore Antichristi* written by Adso of Montier-en-Der about 950.[22] Details from this text were perpetuated endlessly in both the learned and the popular medieval treatises on the Antichrist.

Here is Adso's version of the Antichrist's birth:[23]

> But now let us consider the origin of Antichrist. The source of my information is not my own imagination or invention; rather I found all this in written works after careful research. My authorities say that Antichrist will be born from the tribe of Dan, according to the words of the prophet: "Dan is like a snake by the road side, an adder on the path" [Gen. 49:17]. For he will sit like a serpent by the road side, and he will be on the path to strike those who walk on the paths of righteousness [Ps. 23:3] and kill them with the venom of his malice. He will be born as the result of sexual intercourse of his mother and father,[24] like other men, and not, as some say from a virgin alone. But he will be conceived entirely in sin [Ps. 51:5], he will be engendered in sin, and he will be born in sin [John 9:34]. At the very beginning of his conception, the devil will enter with him into his mother's womb, and by the devil's strength he will be fostered and protected in his mother's womb, and the devil's strength will be with him always.[25] And just as the Holy Ghost came into the womb of the Mother of our Lord Jesus Christ and covered her with his strength and filled her with divinity, so that she conceived from the Holy Ghost and what was born was divine and holy [Luke 1:35]: so also the devil will go down into the womb of Antichrist's mother and fill her completely, possess her completely inside and out, so that she will conceive by man with the devil's assistance, and what is born will be completely foul, completely evil, completely ruined. That is why that man is called the son of destruction [2 Thess. 2:3], because as far as he can he will destroy the human race, and he will himself be destroyed at the Last Judgment.[26] Now you have heard about the manner of his birth; hear also the place where he is to be born. For just as our Lord and Savior preordained Bethlehem for Himself, the place where He put on humanity for us and deigned to be born, so the devil knows a fit place for this man of perdition called Antichrist, whence it is fitting that all evil will arise [1 Tim. 6:10], namely the city of Babylon [Rev. 18:10]. For in this community, which was once a famous and proud

city of the heathen [Isa. 13:19] and the capital of the Kingdom of the Persians, Antichrist will be born.[27] It is said that he will be brought up and live in the towns of Bethsaida and Corozain; for the Lord condemns these towns in the Gospel with the words: "Woe to thee, Corozain, woe to thee, Bethsaida" [Matt. 11:21; Luke 10:13].

Adso's text was widely known and quoted throughout the Middle Ages, because it provided a coherent narrative of the Antichrist's life emphasizing that it was a counterpart to Christ's life. That Adso mentioned three cities as the sites of the Antichrist's birth and childhood caused some confusion and even led later commentators to simply equate Chorozaim and Babylon. Adso's work found its way into one of the most popular spiritual encyclopedias of the Middle Ages, Honorius Augustodensis's *Elucidarium*.[28] Written in Latin in the early twelfth century, this work was translated into many vernacular languages and thus became a veritable storehouse for ideas on every kind of subject, including the life of the Antichrist. A German translation appeared at the end of the twelfth century and for the first time presented the term "Endkrist."[29] "Endkrist" emphasizes the Antichrist's appearance at the end of times, rather than his being the opposite of Christ as implied by the term "Antichrist."[30] Despite the different name, though, Endkrist still figures as both Christ's antitype and imitator in the German vitae.

The *Elucidarium* is set up as a dialogue between a master and his pupil. In answer to the pupil's wish to hear something about the Antichrist, the master proffers the information that the Antichrist was born in Great Babylon of a prostitute of the tribe of Dan. In his mother's womb he was already filled with the devil, and he was raised in Chorozaim by evil sorcerers.[31] The phrase "magna Babylonia" used by Honorius reappears in the captions to the fifteenth-century block books where the Antichrist's birthplace is identified as "Gross Babylon."[32]

One of the most explicit and lurid stories of the Antichrist's birth can be found in Hildegard of Bingen's *Scivias*. Even as a girl the Antichrist's mother is full of all vices. The devil deceives her by acting like an angel and sending her into a kind of desert, where she—unbeknownst to her parents—leads a life of vice and dissolution. Hildegard's terminology reaches a shrill pitch when she describes the conception of the Antichrist; he will be conceived in passionate fornication and his mother will not know who the father is. In a perverted imitation of the Virgin Mary, the Antichrist's mother will then claim that she has known no man and people will believe her claims and call her holy.[33]

Hildegard introduced a strong sexual element into the story of the Antichrist's conception. Before her version in the *Scivias,* the conception itself had not explicitly been viewed as perverse; rather, Adso had insisted on the fact that the Antichrist was conceived by human parents. The perversity had been implied by the devil's "descending" into the mother's uterus. This new tale of sexual license proved very influential. Later texts whose authors claim to use as their source the rather vague text of the *Compendium theologicae* show a clear tendency to embroider upon the sober facts found in the *Compendium.*[34] The exact nature of the relationship of Antichrist to the devil was unclear. The *Compendium* on the one hand described the devil's role in the Antichrist's conception but then, in the following chapter, equated the two.

In a thirteenth-century French play, *Le jour du jugement,* Satan disguises himself as an attractive young man to lie with a young Jewish woman from Babylon, the future mother of the Antichrist.[35] In an unusually explicit scene the mother suffers the pains of pregnancy and complains to a *damoiselle* who is sent to help her. With the aid of "Mahon" (Mohammed) the Antichrist is finally delivered and handed over to the devil for his education. Many details from the learned traditions show up in this convoluted version of the Antichrist's birth. No fewer than four of the manuscript illuminations show the details of the birth: the mother is shown pregnant, then in bed, covered by a blanket, while the *damoiselle* holds the Antichrist in diapers. In the third picture, the mother reaches out toward her baby and in the fourth the child stands on the bed while two devils watch.[36] This mid-fourteenth-century illumination contains one element that becomes prominent in one type of the later German woodcuts: the devils standing around the mother's bed.

The same motif also appears in a manuscript (ca. 1465) of an early-fourteenth-century German text called *Die Erlösung* (the Redemption), which belongs to a different tradition of depicting the Antichrist's birth. The little Antichrist is dark-skinned; his mother is an old woman. The *Jour du jugement* and the *Erlösung* represent some of the other iconographic possibilities available for the depiction of the Antichrist's birth.

Two other texts (one of them illustrated) can be considered as preliminary steps in the formation of the iconographic tradition showing the Antichrist's birth by Caesarean: the Velislaus Bible and Berengier's *De l'avènement Antecrist.* The famous fourteenth-century *Velislai biblia picta* is a fascinating biblical picture book.[37] Of the 747 pen-and-ink drawings, twelve belong to a cycle about the Antichrist. As Karel Stejskal indicates in his introduction, "the literary model for them was found in chapters VII–IX of the work *Compendium totius theologiae veritatis* . . . a popular book in Bohemia." But one crucial element is added to the text of the *Compendium;* in the caption above the picture of the Antichrist's birth (fol. 130) we read: "Nascet autem in babylonia de tribu dan et *erunt diabli obstetrices*" (the devils shall be midwives). The picture indeed shows two devils as midwives: in the center, one holds the swaddled infant in place on top of a low column; on the left, the other stands with outstretched arms at the head of the mother's bed. The guardian angel (soon to be dismissed) stands on the other side. Thus, even though we do not yet see a Caesarean, the devilish midwives have already entered the iconographic pattern of the Antichrist's birth.

But there is another image, on the facing page (fol. 131), that iconographically resembles scenes of Caesarean birth: the Antichrist's circumcision. The circumcision is already mentioned in Haimo of Auxerre's bible commentary[38] and in the *Compendium theologicae,* which provides most of the captions for the *Velislai Bible.* But the text is modified here so that the purpose of the circumcision is no longer the perverse imitation of Christ but simply "to confirm the law of the Jews." The long-haired Antichrist, looking like a woman, is stretched out in a manner reminiscent of many of the Caesarean scenes we studied in Chapter 2. A group of Jews, recognizable by their hats, stands around him; one of them wields a large knife. The place he is aiming for is of course very close to the place where the incision for a Caesarean would be made. The juxtaposition of the birth and circumcision, then, is extremely suggestive and may have led to some kind of iconographic contamination.

Another element shown graphically in the German woodcuts, that of incest between a father and daughter, appears in Berengier's thirteenth-century French version of the Antichrist's birth. Based loosely on Honorius's *Elucidarium,* the *De l'avènement Antecrist* tells of the Antichrist's conception: the mother is not only a prostitute (Honorius's *meretrix*) of the tribe of Dan but also incestuously involved with her father. Berengier contrasts this perverse conception with the virgin birth of our Lord. He also dwells on the perversity of the Antichrist's family relationships: his father is his grandfather, he points out, and his mother is his sister[39]—no wonder, then, that the son grows into a "cruel dragon."

The equation of the Antichrist with a dragon or serpent yields another piece of the Antichrist puzzle. The ninth-century encyclopedist Rabanus

Maurus deals with serpents and the Antichrist in his *De universo*.[40] The quote from Gen. 49:17 provides the basis for a series of resemblances between the viper and the Antichrist. The most important passage for our purposes is the one on the viper's perverse methods of conceiving and giving birth. During the sexual act the male sticks his head into the female's mouth; she bites it off at the moment when the male emits the semen. When the young ones are ready to be born they do so in an unnatural manner: they break through the sides of the mother and thus kill her. As a result, Rabanus concludes, both father and mother die in the act of procreation: the father during conception, the mother during birth. This text formed part of later bestiaries and was known in the vernacular through works like Brunetto Latini's *Livres dou Trésor*.[41] Here, as in Rabanus's text, the voluptuous and libidinous nature of the vipers is stressed. The young vipers are accused of having caused their parents' death. A similar accusation is leveled against Julius Caesar in Jean Mansel's *Histoires romaines* where one of the explanations of the name Caesar reads: "because he killed his mother at birth."[42] Thus a chain of ideas is created that involves unnatural and destructive birth (by splitting open or by incision), the Antichrist-viper and Julius Caesar.

The equation between a Roman emperor and the Antichrist had, of course, been made much earlier in Apocalyptic writings and may have suggested, by a rather circuitous route, the manner of the Antichrist's birth. As in a large number of other texts, the Roman emperors from Nero to Diocletian prefigure the Antichrist in the writings of Otto von Freising.[43] A clear connection between Rome and the Antichrist appears in the twelfth-century German *Ludus de Antichristo,* where the worship demanded by the Antichrist recalls that of the Roman imperial cult. The view of Rome as a new Babylon (the supposed birthplace of the Antichrist) also contributed to the idea of the Antichrist as a Roman emperor. While for some writers, such as Otto, Babylon was the Antichrist's place of origin only in the tropological sense, others took this indication literally.[44] Even Christian Rome was called a new Babylon in the tropological exegesis of 1 Pet. 5:13: "She who is at Babylon . . . sends you greetings."[45] In typological thinking, the Roman emperor most frequently associated with the Antichrist was Nero. Now, Nero had been known for cutting open his mother in order to see where he came from. This cruel action was the subject of many medieval manuscript illuminations that iconographically often resembled images of Caesarean section.

All this diverse material, then, came to form part of both the learned and the popular imagination in the later Middle Ages, and it was from these complex textual and iconographic traditions that a German illustrator of the fifteenth century formed the idea to depict the Antichrist's birth as a Caesarean section.

How closely does a text's illustration follow its contents? We saw in Chapter 2 that often the illustrations are quite independent of the text. For the iconographic tradition of the Antichrist's birth, it seems that the illustrator often functioned as a commentator. His role varied in the three different types of books featuring images of the Antichrist's birth as a Caesarean: block books (or xylographic books), chiroxylographic block books, and printed books. In block books the pages were printed from a single woodblock into which both text and image(s) were carved; text and image were most likely conceived and executed by the same person. In chiroxylographic books the images (and possibly a frame) were printed from a woodblock, while the text was filled in by hand by a scribe. Woodcuts in printed books were set into a page composed of movable type. The design and execution of woodcut illustrations were divided between the *Reisser* and the cutter. The *Reisser* "denotes the designer in relation to a print, strictly speaking the artist who draws with a pen on the block or on paper for transfer to a block."[46] In general, the *Reisser* (possibly in consultation with an overall designer or the author) would be the one to come up with the ideas for the content of a given illustration.

Thus in each category the relationship between text and image was slightly different. Block books are really not so much books as captioned woodcuts bound together. The emphasis is clearly on the image. For block books, image and text were most likely cut by the same person: the illustrator-author, who may have had some guidance from a learned "conceptualizer." For printed books, the illustrator and the scribe or typesetter were most likely not identical. Nevertheless, one can assume that the illustrators read the text.

From these formal considerations some preliminary points emerge. The different layouts in books dealing with the Antichrist indicate that they were meant for different audiences. In block books the pictures tell the story; their layout resembles modern comic books. As Rudolf Hirsch observes, they were mostly bought by "unsophisticated people, of whom many may have been illiterate or semi-literate."[47] In printed books, the illustrations were generally subordinated to the text and one can assume that their audience was more literate.

For the illustrations of the Antichrist's birth this distinction poses some interesting problems: if the illustrators functioned indeed as commentators, how did they translate their "commentaries" for these different target groups? And how can the relationship between the different texts and their illustrations be described? And most important, since the texts themselves do not contain any references to Caesarean birth, how did the illustrators come up with the many variations on this theme?

The idea of the Antichrist's birth as a Caesarean was created in the medieval imagination from many different sources, and one should not look for a single text that inspired its (or others texts') illustrations. Many early manuscripts of the Apocalypse show a trend toward incorporating material into their illustrations that is not present in the texts' narrative lines. Thus many of the metaphors surrounding the Antichrist's life had been brought to life in the illustrations.[48] If he was the "son of destruction" (*filius perditionis*), what better way was there to show his destructiveness from the very beginning of his life than by having him kill his mother simply by being born?

Certain currents of thought can be activated at a given point and become what Gosbert Schüssler calls *bildwirksam*, or iconographically active.[49] This was clearly the case for the Antichrist's birth by Caesarean. The second half of the fifteenth century suddenly saw a proliferation of these images.

The iconographic tradition of the Antichrist's birth by Caesarean shows two principal versions: the satanic version (devils acting as midwives or attendants) represented by figures 22–24, and the obstetrical version (figures 25–27), where there are no obvious clues to any satanic presence. The two versions are distinguished not only by the contents of the illustrations but also by the texts they accompany. Figures 22–24 all come from different versions of the German *Endkrist*, a popular legend drawn from the *Elucidarium* and its translations, the *Compendium theologicae*, and other sources. In these texts, the Antichrist's conception is usually incestuous: a scene showing an elderly man in bed with a young girl often precedes the scene of the Antichrist's birth. The caption indicates that this is a father incestuously wooing his lovely daughter. Of the few details given of his birth the most important is that he was born in

"Great Babylon." This detail is either omitted or modified in the edifying treatise belonging to figures 25 and 27: the *Seelenwurzgarten* (The souls' herb garden). As is explained in the prologue, this text does for the soul what herbs do for the body. Its version of the Antichrist's birth comes from Hildegard of Bingen's *Scivias* and therefore states that the Antichrist was conceived in a desert and born in mock-virgin birth (in an unspecified place). He was raised in the two cursed cities of Chorozaim and Bethsaida. Figure 26 comes from a Latin version of Pseudo-Methodius; here, Antichrist's birthplace is Chorozaim, and Bethsaida is the place where he grew up.

One difference between the two versions emerges from this comparison of the accompanying texts: If the place of the Antichrist's birth is specified as Babylon, as it is in the different versions of the *Endkrist* legend, devils are present at the scene of the Caesarean birth; if the Antichrist's birthplace is given as Chorozaim or remains unspecified, the attendants at the birth are human and, for that matter, nothing in the images suggests that they show the Antichrist's birth and not just any Caesarean birth.

In the earliest representation (fig. 22), from a chiroxylographic block book (ca. 1450), the mother's twisted position suggests physical distress, which contrasts with the serene expression on her face. Her eyes seem to be open, yet they are averted from the child and the satanic midwife (called "bose hebam," evil midwife, in a small caption). This detail immediately creates an intimacy between the devil and the infant; the mother is left out—her function has been fulfilled. In the picture below (on the same page) a very handsome grown-up Antichrist is flirting with two women. Above his head is perched a miniature version of the devilish midwife, a device that is used throughout the text to identify the Antichrist. Women's roles are clearly delineated on this page: they give birth and die, or they become the objects of the Antichrist's lascivious advances.

In figure 22, the mother still seemed to be alive, though on the point of death. In figures 23 and 24, there is no doubt that the mother has just died: a satanic creature is removing a tiny human figure, representing the soul, from the mother's mouth. An angel hovers in the background, ready to receive the soul. The devotional gesture of the soul and the presence of the angel suggest that the mother will be saved and not be blamed for giving birth to the "son of perdition." This is consonant with the *Endkrist* texts, which portray Antichrist's mother as a victim of incestuous seduction. The violent blame and condemnation of the Antichrist's mother on the grounds of her indiscriminate fornication and perverse claims to a virgin birth (evident in such texts as Hildegard's *Scivias*) would, of course, preclude any depiction of salvation.

Unlike in many other images of Caesarean birth, the mothers here are shown fully dressed in flowing robes that are slit in front in the shape of the Caesarean incision.[50] Significantly, no provisions common in other birth scenes (such as a tub with water or a warming fire) have been made for the newborn; instead, monsters stand ready to receive him. This may have been suggested by texts like *Le jour du jugement,* where the mother hands over her newborn Antichrist to the devils by saying: "I should render grace to Mohammed [for the devils' offer of educating the child in their art] / I give him into your care."[51]

The Antichrist is thus shown to be in the hands of the devil (or devils) from the moment of his birth. In the preceding textual traditions, there were many indications that the devil "descended" into the mother's womb after conception. The illustrators translated these indications into dramatic and frightening images. The mother's (physical) "perdition" becomes evident in the fatal Caesarean section; but her spiritual salvation is assured through the angel's presence. Her son is taken from her by satanic midwives and given to equally satanic educators.

The second group of illustrations (fig. 25–27), the obstetrical version, forms a striking contrast to the satanic versions of the birth scene. Here, there are only human attendants and the interior is a tranquil birth chamber. The death of the mother is not dramatized: no small human figure representing the soul escapes from the mother's mouth. Significantly, the obstetrical version did not replace the satanic version but existed alongside it. The two versions, then, are examples of two different types of imagination and inspiration. The obstetrical version appears less explicitly symbolic and more realistic.

The two illustrations from the *Seelenwurzgarten* (figs. 25 and 27) show the undressed mother in bed; she is covered with a cloth up to the point from which the child emerges. This detail alone makes these images more realistic than those in the first group: no Caesarean section could be performed by cutting through a garment. The mother's eyes are closed in figure 25, but open in figure 27. In both pictures she lies motionless. A midwife holds onto the mother's left arm; an attendant gently lifts the child by the shoulders.

The pattern is slightly different in figure 26 (from the Pseudo-Methodius). Unlike in the other pictures, the baby is already delivered here; wrapped in swaddling clothes, he is being cradled by the midwife. She wears the same type of turban as the midwives in figures 25 and 27. Another midwife, or attendant, lurks in the background. While the mothers' faces in the previous illustrations looked rather serene, here her face is contorted; she seems to look at her stomach, slit open in the center. She pays little attention to the newborn, thus underlining, once again, the dissociation of the mother from the birth.

There is no suggestion of the mother's spiritual salvation in these images. In the texts accompanying figures 25 and 27, the *Seelenwurz-garten,* the mother is condemned in the harsh terms used by Hildgard in her *Scivias.* Her death in childbirth may thus be seen as a punishment for her sins. But, at the same time, her early death seems to make her less responsible for her son's future crimes. And what better way to make sure the audience understands that the mother vanishes early on (and thus relinquishes her responsibility) than to show the birth as a Caesarean?

What could have been the audience's reaction to these images? It is possible that the obstetrical version was even more frightening than the satanic version. Does it not show that the Antichrist is "one of us," that he can hide anywhere under normal human features? It seems that this less dramatic approach is more sophisticated and possibly intended for a different type of audience, an audience that can draw its own conclusions. This point is supported by the fact that the obstetrical versions come from printed books (even one Latin text), where the illustrations are more or less subordinated to the text. By contrast, most of the satanic scenes come from block books, whose picture-book layout indicates that they were meant for a less sophisticated audience. Thus, illustrators distinguished between their different target groups: for more sophisticated readers, the commentary was more implicit; the images called for greater capacities of interpretation. For the less sophisticated group, the drama of the Antichrist's birth is spelled out more explicitly. The illustrations leave no doubt as to the devil's direct involvement in the Antichrist's birth. Also, the satanic versions come from texts that explicitly refer to Babylon as the Antichrist's birthplace. It seems, then, that the illustrators who dealt with the primitive captions originating in the *Elucidarium* and the *Compendium theologicae,* created pictures that they saw as especially apt, given the reference to Babylon. In their function as commentators they elucidated the meaning of "Babylon" by including a variety of devils in their pictures. But the obstetrical version was a valid alternative to the satanic one. The crucial point is, of course, that illustrators working for two essentially different audiences chose to depict the Antichrist's birth as a Caesarean. Thus these illustrations reveal how late medieval culture conceived of Caesarean birth: it was seen, by at least one segment of this culture, as profoundly unnatural and destructive and hence worthy of being associated with the Antichrist's birth. The circumstances of his birth differed, but the message sent by the illustrators was the same: whether delivered by human or devilish midwives, the Antichrist is in our midst and ready to seduce even the most faithful.

Caesarean birth was a reality in medieval and Renaissance Europe, but it also formed part of the *imaginaire*. The previous chapters traced the ideas on Caesarean birth in medicine and iconography and studied the roles of midwives or surgeons in the performance of the operation. This chapter has allowed us to place Caesarean birth into both the popular and the learned imagination. For the Antichrist's birth in particular, the two currents interacted and produced a stunning visual representation of the birth of evil. By contrast, the miracles involving Caesarean birth focused on salvation. Since most of the fetuses delivered in these stories were dead, the mothers took center stage and their well-being constituted the essence of the miracle. The miracles dramatized the emergency situation in which most Caesareans take place; they highlighted the skill and devotion of the saintly obstetricians. They also emphasized the importance of a visible mark, the tangible proof of a successful miracle that, in normal childbirth, is absent from the mother's body.

Saintly and satanic obstetricians, then, labored at the same task but with opposite results; while the former were instruments of salvation, the latter delivered evil and damnation. This contrast underlines the twofold nature of Caesarean birth, which we have observed in many different contexts: it encompasses good and evil, life and death, salvation and mutilation.

APPENDIX

CREATIVE ETYMOLOGY:
"CAESAREAN SECTION"
FROM PLINY TO ROUSSET

Although the legend of Caesar's birth by Caesarean was well known in the Middle Ages, no text before the end of the sixteenth century used the term "Caesarean section." When was this term first used in a medical context? Was Julius Caesar really born by Caesarean? And if he was not, where does the term derive from?[1] The association of Julius Caesar with Caesarean section was the result of a long and complicated process of etymological thinking. Medieval etymology was not a historical science; it did not work with phonetic laws, sound shifts, or reconstructive philology. Rather, it was a fundamental way of looking at the world, of making connections and of determining a given term's place in the scheme of things. The immense popularity of Isidore of Seville's *Etymologies* bears witness to the centrality of etymological thought in the Middle Ages.

In grammar and rhetoric, in history, geography, and exegesis, etymological methods were used. Going back to Plato's dialogue *Cratylus* and his ideas on the natural or conventional origins of language, the controversy over the ultimate source of words continued through the Middle Ages and formed an important part of medieval scholarship. Since the Greek word *etymologia* signified the search for truth (in or through words),[2] it was believed that if only the true meaning of a word, especially of a proper name, were known one would have a grasp on the essence of this word, concept, or person. As E. R. Curtius has pointed out, Homer and Pindar indulged in etymological playing with names.[3] In the New Testament, authorization for the interpretation of names can be found in Matt. 16:18, where Jesus calls Peter the rock on which the church will be built (Latin *petra*, "rock"). The etymological exploration of names as an exegetical technique became especially important in the works of Saint Jerome (for example, the *Liber de nominibus hebraicis*) as well as in those of Saint Augustine. Curtius quotes Augustine's play on the name of Paulus, supposedly named this way because he was the "minimus apostolorum," or the smallest of the apostles (Latin *paulus*, "small"; *minimus*, "the smallest").[4]

For many medieval scholars a close relationship existed between etymology and genealogy. Founding myths, for example, were often closely linked to proper names of historical or mythological figures. Thus Britain supposedly got its name from Brutus, one of Aeneas's descendants; the German town Jülich was said to derive its name from its founding father Julius Caesar. Examples of this kind could be multiplied endlessly. The etymological relationship between a name and its supposed source was such a common literary proceeding that it was expressed in certain formulas, such as *nomen habet a* (it gets the name from . . .) or in Old French *de ceo vint li nuns* (the name comes from this . . .), a set expression found countless times in Wace's *Roman de Brut* (ca. 1150), which deals with the settlement of Britain by Trojan refugees. The faith in etymological explanations as a way to gain a more perfect knowledge of a given idea was thus fundamental to the medieval imagination and it was this faith that helped entrench the idea of Julius Caesar's Caesarean birth.

Before tracing the different stages of this entrenchment we must address one further preliminary question: Why were multiple etymologies so popular? Was not etymology a means to recover one ultimate signification? In exegesis, it was believed that God as the ultimate Word had created univocal significations at the beginning of time. For late antique and medieval exegetes, the current multiplicity of tongues and races represented a fall from grace. As Howard Bloch points out, "both history and grammar are bound by a common sense of loss and dispersion, by a common nostalgic longing for beginnings, and by a set of ontologically similar strategies of return."[5] The conflict between linguistic determinism (the nostalgia for univocal meaning) and "the intellectual awareness of the socially determined nature of language" could not be resolved.[6] Multiple etymologies find their place at the heart of this conflict: faith in the possibility of a return to the perfect one-ness collided with a passion for exhaustive research.[7] For the etymology of "Caesarean section" legendary and medical material coalesced to form a complex web of ideas.

One possible derivation of the term "Caesarean section" is from the phrase *lex caesarea,* which may have come from a renaming of the *lex regia,* or royal law, dating from approximately 715 B.C. This law, proclaimed under King Numa Pompilius, stated that it was unlalwful to bury a pregnant woman without attempting to cut out the child in order to save its life.[8] Supposedly this law was rebaptized *lex caesarea* under the first Roman emperor, Caesar Augustus, Julius Caesar's adopted son. As intriguing as this suggestion is—establishing as it does a link between the law and Julius Caesar's family—neither the term itself nor its renaming is attested beyond doubt.[9] The connection that was made between the two terms thus illustrates certain ways of (wishful) etymological thinking rather than any real historical development.

The most durable derivation of the name Caesar proved to be the one from *caesus,* "cut," first mentioned by Pliny the Elder (A.D. 23–79) in his *Natural History:* "Auspicatius enecta parente gignuntur, sicut Scipio Africanus prior natus, primusque Caesarum a caeso matris utero dictus, qua de causa et Caesones appellati. Simili modus natus est Manilium qui Carthaginem cum exercitu intravit" (It is a better omen when the mother dies in giving birth to the child; instances are the birth of the elder Scipio Africanus and of the first of the Caesars, who got that name from the surgical operation performed on his mother; the origin of the family named Caeso is also the same. Also Manilius who entered Carthage with his army was born in the same manner).[10] This ambiguous passage caused many misunderstandings that had a direct influence on the development of the legend concerning Caesar's birth as well as on the extraordinary iconographic tradition that resulted from this legend. The persistent, but most productive, misreading of Pliny's text hinged on the question of the identity of this "first of the Caesars." Was he Scipio Africanus? The passage just cited could certainly be interpreted this way. Or does "primusque Caesarum" refer to another member of the *gens Julia* bearing the surname Caesar (as one entire branch of the family did)? But if so, which one? Pliny provided no clear-cut answer.

After Pliny, the surname Caesar continued to preoccupy various commentators for whom the problem of the manner of birth evoked by "Caesar" constituted but one problem among many. At the end of the third century, for example, Aelius Spartianus considered the etymological origin of "Caesar" in a letter to the emperor Diocletian. He grouped together four possibilities which—either together or separately—remained in vogue throughout the entire medieval period: (1) one of the

Caesars, most likely the first to bear this surname, Sextus Julius Caesar, who was praetor in 208 B.C., killed an elephant (in Punic, *caesar*) during the second Punic war (218–201);[11] (2) the first Caesar was cut from his mother's womb after her death (Aelius does not specify here which member of the family of the Caesars he has in mind); (3) one of the early Caesars was born with a big shock of hair (*caesaries*, from Sanskrit, *Kéçah*); or (4) he was born with bluish green eyes (Latin *caesius*, blue-green). The first possibility is well attested through the existence of Roman coins showing Julius Caesar on one side and an elephant on the other, thus commemorating his ancestor's exploit.[12]

The grammarian Sextus Pompeius Festus, who flourished sometime in the first four centuries A.D., distinguished between those born by Caesarean, who are called *caesones,* and the possible reason for Caesar's gaining this surname, his abundant hair: "Caesones appellantur ex utero matris exsecti; Caesar, quod est cognomen Juliorum, a caesarie dictus est, quia scillicet cum caesarie natus est" (*Caesones* are called those who have been cut out of the mother's womb; *Caesar,* which is the surname of the Julians, comes from *caesaries* [a lot of hair] because he was born with much hair). Pompeius Festus's work reached the Middle Ages through an abridgment by Paul the Deacon (720?–799?) and thus played a role in the transmission of two of the etymological possibilities also envisaged by Aelius Spartianus: the abundant hair and the operation of cutting.

Isidore of Seville (ca. 570–636) in his *Etymologies,* characterized by Howard Bloch as a work where we find "the recuperation of all philosophy by grammar, and even . . . a lexicology which takes on metaphysical proportions", made the definitive and unequivocal connection between Julius Caesar and Caesarean birth: "Caesar autem dictus, quod caeso mortuae matris utero prolatus eductusque fuerit, vel quia cum caesarie natus sit. A quo imperatores sequentes Caseares dicti, eo quod comati essent. Qui enim execto utero eximebantur, Caesones et Caesares appellabantur."[13] Thus Isidore restricted himself to two possibilities for the origin of Caesar's surname: he was called Caesar because he was cut from his dead mother's womb or because he was born with abundant hair. Isidore then goes on to a general application of his explanation. The principal purpose of this passage was to explain why Roman rulers were called Caesars, but in the process Isidore succeeded in linking once and for all Caesarean birth to Julius Caesar. It was through this text, then, that the idea of Caesar's birth by Caesarean section was perpetuated and entered vernacular literature.

Isidore's version of Caesar's birth was used at the beginning of a widely read compilation and translation of Roman historians, the anonymous *Faits des Romains,* written in French prose in the early thirteenth century: "Gaius Juilles Cesar fu tant eu vantre sa mere que il covint le ventre tranchier et ovrir ainz que il en poist oissir; et trova l'en que il avoit mout granz chevex. Por ce fu il apelez Cesar par sornon, car cist moz Cesar puet senefier ou chevelure ou trenchement" (Gaius Julius Caesar was so long in his mother's belly that one had to cut open the belly so that he could come out; and one found that he had a lot of hair. Therefore one gave him the surname Caesar, for this word Caesar can mean hair or cutting).[14] Thus the *Faits des Romains,* by incorporating and translating Isidore's version of Caesar's birth, made it available to a very large vernacular audience.

The early years of Caesar's life as narrated in the *Faits* are based on Suetonius's (A.D. 69–140) *The Twelve Caesars.* But as the first sections of Suetonius's text were lost, the author of the *Faits* had to find another source: Isidore. The conquest of Gaul in the *Faits,* as well, is not re-counted according to Suetonius but according to Caesar's *De bello gallico. The Twelve Caesars* was also known independently in this period, not only as a source for the *Faits;* in fact, it was a staple of the medieval classroom. It is in this text that we find a passage that added to the confusion of medieval historiographers who had to deal with Caesar's life. In part 26 of his chapter on Caesar, Suetonius describes Caesar's conquest of Gaul. "During these nine years," we learn, "Caesar lost, one after the other, his mother, his daughter, and his grandson."[15] Now, it was clear to most historiographers that a woman did not survive a Caesarean section. How, then, could one reconcile the version of Caesar's birth found in Isidore and the *Faits* with the late death of Caesar's mother mentioned in Sueto-nius (who relied on Caesar's own testimony in *De bello gallico*)? The solutions found to this problem by one medieval translator, most likely Jean du Chesne, merit close study, as they can be seen as paradigmatic for much of medieval historiography when we are presented with different versions of one event (based on conflicting yet authoritative sources) and are asked to choose the one most convincing to us.[16] Jean du Chesne was commissioned by the Burgundian duke Charles the Bold to translate Caesar's *De bello gallico,* also known as the *Commentaries.* Jean was from Lille in Flanders and came to lead a very productive professional life at the court of Burgundy. For his translation of Caesar's text he used not only the Latin original and other texts, such as Geoffrey of Monmouth's

Historia regum britanniae, but also his topographical knowledge of the regions where Caesar led his campaigns. He can thus be described as a learned clerk, and his relatively wide knowledge of Latin texts of this period explains some of the remarkable passages concerning Caesar's birth that we find in his translation. Since Caesar himself did not speak of his birth in the *Commentaries,* Jean found other sources for this event, one of them the *Faits,* as Flutre and Bossuat have shown.[17]

In one of the manuscripts of Jean's French translation of the *Commentaries,* two of the by now familiar possibilities for the origin of the surname Caesar are listed: the manner of birth and the abundant hair (both based on the *Faits*).[18] The translator is inclined to believe Isidore, that Caesar was born by Caesarean section, rather than Suetonius. According to Jean, Suetonius blamed Isidore (obviously a chronological impossibility) for the false story of Caesar's birth and called it apocryphal (*appocriffe,* fol. 43v), since Caesar lost his mother by natural causes during the campaign in Gaul. The chronological confusion of these two authors is not unusual in the Middle Ages: since both Suetonius and Isidore were considered *auctores* who belonged to the established school curriculum, they were grouped together in "antiquity" without any concern for their real dates of birth. This is why Jean can assert blithely that Suetonius objected to Isidore's definitions of the term "Caesar." As for Caesar's abundant hair, Jean tells us that Suetonius insisted on Caesar's baldness, a condition that he apparently greatly disliked. In fact, Caesar's imperial ambitions were closely related to his baldness: as emperor he would no longer have to uncover his head and no one would notice his lack of hair. Maybe, Jean adds, he was called Caesar (meaning "having abundant hair") in jest, as one often calls people by a nickname designating the opposite of their real qualities or appearance. Or maybe the woman who died when Caesar was an adult was his *mère de lait* (wet nurse). In any case, Caesar had brought his baldness upon himself by walking around bareheaded during his youth and exposing his hair to rain and to heat. And so forth. This type of disconnected musing on the surname Caesar is a striking but by no means unusual example of the medieval translator's method. A digressive style of this sort reflects a certain insecurity in face of (textual) authority; rather than choosing between different versions, Jean lists all of them and even invents some more, thus displaying his erudition and at the same time avoiding the critical stance required in a later age of "critical editions."[19]

An ingenious version of Caesar's birth presenting the two most popular etymological possibilities can be found in the early-fourteenth-century *Roman de Renart le Contrefait,* another poem that relied heavily on the *Faits* for the parts dealing with Julius Caesar:

> Avant que Julius fu nez,
> Sa mere ouvrir l'enconvint;
> Aultrement sur terre ne vint,
> Car trop grant cheveulx il avoit,
> Et pour ce naistre il ne pouvoit.
> Et pour ce Cezar l'appellerent,
> Que pour lui sa mere soierent.
> Cezar, a droitte parleure,
> Signifie chevelure;
> Cezar si est detrenchement,
> Qui bien parle proprement.[20]

(Before Julius was born one had to open up his mother; otherwise he could not come to this earth [i.e., be born] for he had too much hair, and this is why he could not be born. For this reason he is called Caesar, because for him they cut open his mother. Caesar really means "hair"; Caesar means "cutting open", according to those who speak properly.)

This passage illustrates the popularity of the rhetorical figure known as *etymologia* and the creative uses etymology could be put to. The paratactic listing of possibilities characteristic of antique and medieval commentators is complemented here by a narrative sequence connecting the two meanings of the word "Caesar." In the *Roman de Renart le Contrefait,* a monumental work of encyclopedic character, the adventures of Renart are often a mere pretext for theological and philosophical excurses. It is therefore fitting that this passage exhibits, *en miniature* as it were, techniques typical for the work as a whole. The treatment of etymology here, integrated as it is into a narrative framework, contrasts markedly with the above-cited involved passage on Caesar's birth offered by Jean du Chesne 150 years later. The contrasting aim and methods of a poet (the author of the *Renart*) and Jean as chronicler-translator can be illustrated through the juxtaposition of the two passages describing Caesar's birth: where one aims for narrative coherence, the other is content to list a whole series of etymological and legendary traditions without worrying about truth or logic. The author of the *Roman de Renart le Contrefait* also was a clerk, of course, but he used knowledge that formed part of the learned canon of the period and made it part of a narrative; or, as Emile Benveniste has shown in a different context, succession or sequence is transformed into causality.[21] Both of these texts, then, are striking examples of what can best be described as creative etymology.

The works I have discussed so far all made reference to Isidore and his remarks on the etymology of the surname Caesar. In one of the later translations of Roman history, Jean Mansel's *Histoires romaines,* written in 1454, we again find the *Faits* version of Caesar's birth, this time, however, attributed to Lucan.[22] Here is the text according to manuscript Arsenal 5088 (my transcription): "Pour ce que dorenanvant sera souvent parlé de Gayus Julius cesar et de ses fais qui furent haulz et merveilleux, Il couvient ensieuvir en ceste partie lucan qui plus a plain en traitte que nul autre" (Because we will now speak often of Julius Caesar and his deeds, which were noble and marvellous, we have to follow for this part Lucan, who deals more explicitly with this than anyone else [fol. 43v]). The sentence from the *Faits* (quoted above) describing Caesar's birth follows. Now, it is true, that Lucan was one of the sources for the *Faits* (although his text underwent an ideological transformation necessitated by the positive image of *Caesar* in the *Faits*). But Lucan most certainly did not mention Caesar's birth. It is clear, then, from Jean Mansel's text that the account of Caesar's birth in the *Faits* had attached itself so firmly to Caesar's name that no history of Caesar would be complete without it.[23] There is no doubt that the *Faits* constituted the authoritative version of Caesar's life (and consequently of his birth) and that the responsibility of making abdominal delivery a truly "Caesarean" birth—and of creating the extraordinarily fertile iconographic tradition—lies with this text.

The strength and persistence of one of the etymological explanations of Caesar's name can be further illustrated through an Arabic manuscript of al-Bīrūnī's *Chronology of Ancient Nations.* In a fourteenth-century manuscript of this eleventh-century text we see a striking depiction of Caesar's birth.[24] Four bearded men attend to a woman stretched out naked and presumably dead. One of the men carefully pulls out the baby through a large incision that spans the entire width of the woman's abdomen. The caption above the picture reads: " . . . and he is called Caesar because his mother died at the time of delivery and her belly was cut open and he was taken out."[25] This statement, probably based on Isidore, does not make much sense in Arabic if the Latin word *caesus* (cut) is not supplied. However, this caption presupposes a familiarity with both Latin etymology and the story of Caesar's birth that is striking for the eleventh century.

Two other versions of Caesar's birth (dating from the thirteenth century) deserve mention. One is in the *Prosa histórica* of Alfonso the Wise, the other in a Catalan chronicle called *Flos mundi*.[26] Alfonso's history offers five different explanations for the name Caesar: (1) the manner of his birth; (2) his abundant hair; (3) because he inaugurated the habit of cutting one's hair; (4) because in his early youth he killed an elephant; (5) because he killed so many enemies (*cedere* [to strike, to kill]).[27] Reasons (3) and (5) have not so far appeared in our survey. They attest to a desire for the picturesque and for the pseudo-logical that we find in the *Roman de Renart le Contrefait* a century later. The last reason, for example, clearly built on the tradition of Caesar as a military leader and conqueror, as it could be found in the *Faits* and the almost contemporary *Histoire ancienne jusqu'à César,* texts certainly known to Alfonso.[28]

Other, even more farfetched reasons for Caesar's name can be found in the *Flos mundi*. The author constructs a whole story around Caesar's birth: one day in Rome, during some sort of skirmish, a woman was killed. A knight noticed that she was pregnant, cut her open, and saved the child. As this happened in the month of July, the child was given the name Julius, and because both his parents were killed that day he was called Caesar. This last explanation relies on the connections between *cedere* (to kill) and Caesar. According to Arturo Graf, who reports this curious episode in his book on the role of Rome in the medieval imagination, this is an example of the creativity of popular (as well as erudite) fantasy, which invented singular and marvelous origins for great men.[29] The two passages just discussed also illustrate the principle of accretion to which most legends are subject. As the figure of Caesar took shape over the medieval period and captured the public's imagination, the legend acquired new and "plausible" elements, such as the dramatization of Caesar's valor reflected in the new connection of *cedere* and "Caesar."

The preoccupation with the possible connections between Julius Caesar and Caesarean section was not limited to areas in which a Romance language was spoken. The German term for Caesarean section, *Kaiserschnitt* (*Kaiser,* "emperor"; *Schnitt,* "incision"), grew out of similar speculations and fabulations, as did the term *opération césarienne,* coined by the Parisian surgeon François Rousset in 1581.

One interesting association of abdominal delivery with an emperor, or *Kaiser,* can be found in a German obstetrical text of the third quarter of the fifteenth century.[30] It is a German version of Latin commentaries on the pseudo-Albertus Magnus's *Secreta mulierum.* In chapter eight (on birth) the author describes a Caesarean section and ends by saying: "und das man die frucht auss der muter leybe solle schneyden als der Erst kaiser hainrich genant kaiser hainrich [*sic*] der wart auss der muter leybe geschnitten" (and one should cut the fruit from the mother's body, as was cut from his mother's body the first emperor Heinrich, called the emperor Heinrich). One could assume from this statement that the text refers to the emperor Heinrich I, who was elected emperor in 919 and reigned till 936. He is the only person that could possibly be designated as the first emperor Heinrich. A look at his life, though, reveals not one detail that could associate him with a birth by Caesarean section.[31] The origin of this mysterious passage must lie elsewhere, most likely in the realm of the imagination. The new fantasy associating the emperor Heinrich with the operation reveals the close connection that must have existed in medieval authors' minds between surgical birth and the idea of "emperor." Heinrich was probably closer to the heart of the German commentator than Julius Caesar, and this is why Heinrich I gets the credit for the naming of the operation.

But the legend of Julius Caesar's birth was well known in Germany and provided a valid alternative explanation for the imperial association of the operation, as can be seen from a passage in Eucharius Roesslin's *Der Swangern Frawen und Hebammen Rosegarten* (1513) in which the author speaks of cases where the mother dies before delivery and the child may still be alive. The midwife is advised to make an incision in the mother's abdomen and to pull out the child. Immediately after this we read: "Also lesen wir in d'römer geschichten das der erst keiser Julius genant von seiner muoter leib geschnitten wart" (We read in the histories [or stories] of the Romans that the first emperor, called Julius, was cut from his mother's body).[32] Thus Roesslin opts for the version that sees the originator of the term in Julius Caesar.

The passages from the pseudo-Albertus Magnus and Roesslin illustrate several popular misconceptions of the medieval period: that Julius Caesar was the first Roman emperor; that he was born by Caesarean section; and that the emperor Heinrich I was born in the same manner and gave the operation its name. Here is one more proof, then, for both the firm hold etymological thinking had on medieval minds and for the creativity this thinking could lead to.

How, then, did the term Caesarean section enter medical terminology? The traditions I have just traced explain the persistent association of

Julius Caesar with this operation. Although some chroniclers expressed doubts about his birth, these were clearly not strong or convincing enough to destroy the legend of Caesar's birth. It is therefore not surprising that the earliest medical writers treating the operation perpetuated this idea. But whereas Bernard of Gordon, when speaking of abdominal delivery in his 1305 *Lilium medicinae* cites Pliny's vague reference to the "first of the Caesars," Guy de Chauliac in his 1363 *Chirurgie* boldly states "Thus Caesar was extracted, as one reads in the histories of the Romans."[33] Most likely, the "histories of the Romans" designate the *Faits*, and not Pliny, as some historians have believed. In 1513, as we saw above, this passage was translated word for word into German by Eucharius Roesslin, who thus transported the idea of Julius Caesar's birth by Caesarean into German territory. None of these authors used the term Caesarean section, however.

It was François Rousset who was responsible for the permanent entrenchment of the term "Caesarean section" in medical terminology. In the dedication to the reader ("Au Lecteur") of his 1581 treatise *Traitté nouveau de l'hystérotomotokie, ou enfantement caesarien,* Rousset states that he "baptized" the operation *opération césarienne.* Since Rousset wrote this treatise in French (a choice that was unusual and needed some justification) and at a time when the French language was receptive to neologisms, his term entered the French vocabulary immediately and permanently. Why did the term "Caesarean section" become permanently associated with Julius Caesar, although Rousset went back to Pliny's possible identification of the "first of the Caesars" as Scipio Africanus? Several facts may account for this: all through the Middle Ages Julius Caesar had been one of the most popular heroes; given the auspicious nature of a Caesarean birth as described by Pliny, it is not too surprising that such a hero should be singled out for a special fate by the wondrous nature of his birth. Another factor was the far-reaching and influential textual and iconographic tradition of the *Faits des Romains,* which left no doubt as to the details of Caesar's birth.

Thus Rousset's term seemed to sanction the long-standing popular and learned association of Julius Caesar with the Caesarean section, an association that led to much confusion concerning the true nature of Caesar's birth.[34] Although ultimately misleading, "Caesarean section"—more picturesque and evocative than most medical terms—proved to be a most enduring contribution to Western medical terminology.

ANNOTATED LIST
OF ILLUSTRATIONS

Pertinent bibliographical references for the illustrations are given in parentheses. "Flutre no." refers to the numbers in L.-F. Flutre's *Les Manuscrits des "Faits des Romains."* All references in abbreviated form are keyed to the Bibliography. For the diffusion and interdependence of manuscripts of the *Faits des Romains,* see Wyss, *Die Caesarteppiche,* and Guénée, "La culture historique des nobles."

Fig. 1: John of Arderne, *Speculum flebotomiae.* Glasgow, Glasgow University Library, MS Hunter 112 (14th–15th cents.), fol. 94r (MacKinney, *Medical Illustrations,* p. 128, no. 66.5). By permission of Glasgow University Library.

Fig. 2: *Les Faits des Romains.* Paris, Bibliothèque Nationale (henceforth B.N.), f. fr. 251 (2d quarter of 14th cent.), fol. 215r (Flutre P5). Phot. Bibl. Nat. Paris. By permission of the Bibliothèque Nationale, Paris.

Fig. 3: *Les Faits des Romains.* Princeton, Princeton University Library, MS Garrett 128 (14th cent.), fol. 144r (*Princeton University Library Chronicle,* 27.3 [Spring 1966], 186–90). Published with permission of Princeton University Library.

Fig. 4: *Les Faits des Romains.* Paris, B.N. f. fr. 23083 (Paris, Honoré style, late 13th cent.), fol. 1r (Flutre P17). Phot. Bibl. Nat. Paris. By permission of the Bibliothèque Nationale, Paris.

Fig. 5: *Les Faits des Romains.* Paris, B.N. n. acq. fr. 3576 (14th cent.), fol. 197r (Flutre P19). Phot. Bibl. Nat. Paris. By permission of the Bibliothèque Nationale, Paris.

Fig. 6: *Les Faits des Romains.* Paris, B.N. f. fr. 246 (1364), fol. 158r (Flutre P3). Phot. Bibl. Nat. Paris. By permission of the Bibliothèque Nationale, Paris.

Fig. 7: *Les Faits des Romains.* London, British Library, Royal MS G 16 VII (14th cent.), fol. 219r (Flutre L1). By permission of the British Library.

Fig. 8: *Les Faits des Romains.* Copenhagen, Kongelige Bibliotek, MS Thott 431 (2d quarter of 14th cent.), fol. 224r (6 × 6 cm) (Flutre H). By permission of the Department of Manuscripts, The Royal Library, Copenhagen.

Fig. 9: *Les Faits des Romains,* ca. 1375, fol. 199r. This manuscript is listed in MacKinney, *Medical Illustrations* (no. 47.1), as Dublin, Chester Beatty Library MS 74. It was painted by Jean Bondol for either Charles V or Jean duc de Berry. (See R. S. Wieck, *Late Medieval and Renaissance Illuminated Manuscripts in the Houghton Library* no. 1). Photograph courtesy of H. P. Kraus, New York. Reproduction courtesy of the Schöyen Collection.

Fig. 10: *Les Faits des Romains.* Brussels, Bibliothèque Royale Albert I, MS 9104–05 (14th cent.), fol. 218r (Flutre B2). Reproduced by permission.

Fig. 11: *Les Faits des Romains.* Venice, Biblioteca Nazionale Marciana, Cod. Marc. Fr. z.3 (14th cent.), fol. 2r (Flutre M). See also Domenico Ciampoli, *I codici francesi della R. Biblioteca Nazionale* (Venezia: Leo S. Olschki, 1897), pp. 6ff. Reproduced by permission.

Fig. 12: *Les Faits des Romains.* Paris, Bibliothèque de l'Arsenal, MS 5186 (15th cent.), fol. 1r (Flutre A). Phot. Bibl. Nat. Paris. By permission of the Bibliothèque Nationale, Paris.

Fig. 13: *Les Faits des Romains.* London, British Library, Royal MS 17 F II (1470), fol. 9r (Flutre L2). By permission of the British Library.

Fig. 14: Julius Caesar, *Commentaires,* trans. Jean du Chesne. London, British Library, Royal MS 16 G VIII (Lille, 1473), fol. 32r. (For the text, see Bossuat, "Traductions françaises".) By permission of the British Library.

Fig. 15: Julius Caesar, *Commentaires,* trans. Jean du Chesne. London, British Library, MS Egerton 1065 (15th cent.), fol. 9r. By permission of the British Library.

Fig. 16: Julius Caesar, *Commentaires,* trans. Jean du Chesne. Oxford, Bodleian Library, MS Douce 208, fol. 1r. Painted by the Bruges Master of 1483. (Cf. Delaissé, *Miniature flamande,* no. 247.) By permission of the Bodleian Library, Oxford.

Fig. 17: *Les Faits des Romains.* Paris, B.N. f. fr. 64 (15th cent.), fol. 234r. Painted by a student of Fouquet (Porcher, *Manuscrits à peintures,* no. 261, p. 126; Flutre P2; Imbault-Huart, *Médecine médiévale,* no. 54, pp. 126–27). Phot. Bibl. Nat. Paris. By permission of the Bibliothèque Nationale, Paris.

Fig. 18: Jean Mansel, *Histoires romaines.* Paris, Bibliothèque de l'Arsenal, MS 5088 (15th cent.), fol. 43r. Painted in the atelier of Liédet (Delaissé, *Miniature flamande,* pp. 72–73; for the text, Flutre, *Li Faits des Romains*). Phot. Bibl. Nat. Paris. By permission of the Bibliothèque Nationale, Paris.

Fig. 19: *Les Faits des Romains.* Paris, B.N. f. fr. 20312 bis (Flemish, 2d half of 15th cent.), fol. 1r (Flutre P15). Phot. Bibl. Nat. Paris. By permission of the Bibliothèque Nationale, Paris.

Fig. 20: Jean Mansel, *Histoires romaines.* Paris, B.N. f. fr. 54 (16th cent.), fol. 258r. Phot. Bibl. Nat. Paris. By permission of the Bibliothèque Nationale, Paris.

Fig. 21: *Miscellaneous Medical Texts.* London, Wellcome Library of the History of Medicine, MS 49 (The Wellcome Apocalypse), (15th cent.), fol. 38v (Kurz, "Medical Illustrations," p. 141). By permission of the Wellcome Institute Library, London.

Fig. 22: *Endkrist.* Chiroxylographic block book in the collection of Otto Schäfer, Schweinfurt (Nuremberg, ca. 1450), fol. 2v (Schreiber, *Handbuch,* 11:52ff.; facsimile by Musper). Courtesy of Bibliothek Otto Schäfer and Prestel Verlag, Munich.

Fig. 23: Entkrist. Block book. Munich, Bayerische Staatsbibliothek, Xyl. 1 (Swabia, mid-15th cent.), fol. 2r (facsimile by Pfister; Schreiber, *Handbuch,* vol. 4; Friedländer, *Der Holzschnitt,* p. 26; Kristeller, *Kupferstich,* p. 37). Reproduced by permission.

Fig. 24: El libro del Anticristo. Zaragoza: Paul Hurus, 1496. Fol. 5. New York Public Library, *KB +1496. (Gesamtkatalog der Wiegendrucke* no. 2058; Goff A-770. The same woodcut was first used in *Entkrist* [Strasbourg, ca. 1482]. *Gesamtkatalog der Wiegendrucke,* no. 2050; facsimile by Kelchner; a more recent facsimile and commentary in Boveland, Burger, and Steffen). By permission of Rare Books and Manuscripts Division, The New York Public Library, Astor, Lenox and Tilden Foundations.

Fig. 25: Seelenwurzgarten. Nuremberg: Fritz Creussner, 1473 (without illustrations); Ulm: Dinckmut, 1483. PML 199 Ch L f 490, fol. dd6v, The Pierpont Morgan Library, New York. (Goff, S-364. There are several later editions of this work.) Reproduced by permission.

Fig. 26: Pseudo-Methodius, *Opusculum divinarum revelationum.* Edited by Sebastian Brant. Basel: Michael Furter, 1504. New York Public Library, Stuart *KB 1504. (Goff M-524. Woodcut repeated in many later editions.) By permission of Rare Books and Manuscripts Division, The New York Public Library, Astor, Lenox and Tilden Foundations.

Fig. 27: Seelenwurzgarten. Augsburg: Schönsperger, 1484. RB 101792, Huntington Library. (Goff S-366.) Reproduced by permission of The Huntington Library, San Marino, California.

NOTES

Abbreviations

BHM	*Bulletin of the History of Medicine*
B.L.	British Library, London
B.N.	Bibliothèque Nationale, Paris
cod.	codex
col.	column
f. fr.	fonds français
fig.	figure
f. lat.	fonds latin
fol.	folio
JHM	*Journal of the History of Medicine and Allied Sciences*
MS	manuscript
n. acq. fr.	nouvelles acquisitions françaises
PL	*Patrologiae cursus completus.* Series latina. Ed. J. P. Migne. Paris, 1844–1864.
r	recto
v	verso

Introduction

1. "Inde Lichan ferit, exsectum iam matre perempta et tibi, Phoebe, sacrum, casus evadere ferri quod licuit parvo" (*Aeneid* 10.315–17). I quote the translation by Allen Mandelbaum (New York: Bantam Books, 1971), p. 254. For the history of the term "Caesarean section," see the Appendix.

2. The story of this child, later to become abbot of Saint Gall, contains these details: "[The mother's] time drew near; she fell into a sore sickness before her time, and died a fortnight before the expected birth. The child was cut from her corpse and wrapped in the

fat of a new-born pig, until his skin should grow. . . . The boy, who was most comely, was delicately nurtured in the abbey. The brethren called him 'The Unborn'; and seeing that his birth was thus untimely, and that no fly ever bit him without drawing blood, therefore in his case the master spared even the rod." The combination of these two privileges is mysterious, but it indicates that those born by Caesarean are singled out for special treatment by both humans and animals. It may be that the fly's behavior marked the abbot as physically different. In any case, the surname "Unborn" forever signaled the abbot's essential otherness through his unnatural birth; not only was he not born in the natural manner, but he was cut from a corpse. See Coulton, *Life in the Middle Ages,* 4:80–81. The Latin text is in Goldast, *Rerum alamannicarum scriptores,* p. 40. The detail about the fly's bite does not appear in any other stories about people born by Caesarean.

3. This is why Shakespeare could, in *Macbeth,* play on the prophecy that "none of woman born / Shall harm Macbeth" (act 4, sc. 1). This prophecy becomes the central enigma in the tragedy and is at last ironically fulfilled when Macduff informs Macbeth that "Macduff was from his mother's womb / Untimely ripp'd" (act 5, sc. 8). Significantly, Shakespeare changed the scene of the prophecy from that in his source, Holinshed. In Holinshed it was a witch who prophesied that Macbeth "should never be slaine with man born of anie woman" (Boswell-Stone, *Shakespeare's Holinshed,* p. 36). In *Macbeth,* the apparition of a bloody child makes a similar pronouncement. Shakespeare's picture of Caesarean birth was therefore both realistic and symbolic. The bloodiness of the operation, represented by the child, is, in this scene, tied to its symbolic and mysterious dimensions.

4. Given the conditions of the times, it must be assumed that the mother died during the birth. See Glesinger, "La Naissance de Vopiscus Fortunatus Plempius," p. 678.

5. Cf. Brody, *The Disease of the Soul.*

6. For discussion of these questions as they relate to present-day women, see Sandra Blakeslee, "Doctors Debate Surgery's Place in the Maternity Ward" (*New York Times,* March 24, 1985); Tamar Lewin, "Courts Acting to Force Care of Unborn" (*New York Times,* November 23, 1987); Philip Shabecoff, in "Panel Says Caesareans Are Used Too Often" (*New York Times,* November 3, 1987), states that 24.1 percent of all births in 1986 were Caesareans. The rate has quadrupled over the last sixteen years. Sandra Blakeslee quotes one doctor as saying, "You rarely get sued for doing a C-section. It's easier to tell the jury, 'I did everything I could. I did an immediate C-section.'" The preference for C-sections may also be related to class. Blakeslee points out that 80 percent of well-to-do Brazilian women deliver by Caesarean. For a judicious evaluation of the pros and cons of Caesarean birth (focusing also on Brazil), see Marlise Simons, "Babies and Doctors: Whose Birth Is It Anyway?" (*New York Times,* July 5, 1988). On the rights of mothers and fetuses, see Marcia Chambers, "Are Fetal Rights Equal to Infants'?" (*New York Times,* November 16, 1986).

7. Several characters in legend and literature were born by Caesarean, all of them male. (The birth of female babies is usually not described in great detail.) In eleventh-century Iran, the poet Firdusi told of the birth of the hero Rustam by Caesarean section in a moving passage of his *Shahnama.* See Torpin and Vafaie, "The Birth of Rustam." In the medieval European tradition, Tristan (in the late-twelfth-century German version of *Tristan* by Eilhart) was born by Caesarean on a sea journey. The birth here predicts Tristan's dark future and can be seen as a metaphor for the destructive forces governing man's fate from the moment of his birth. Both Rustam's (= "I am relieved of suffering") and Tristan's ("triste" = sad [for the mother's death]) names commemorate the manner of their birth. A medieval Scandinavian ballad, *The Death of Queen Dagmar,* also tells of a royal Caesarean birth fatal to the mother. Here paradise is the reward for the mother's sufferings. See Jacobsen, "Pregnancy and Childbirth," p. 98. In the mythological tradition, the births of Aesculapius, Adonis, and Bacchus are Caesareans. Some interesting inter-

pretations of these births can be found in the fourteenth-century Christianized moraliza-
tion of Ovid's *Metamorphoses,* the 72,000-line *Ovide moralisé.* Generally, Caesarean birth is
seen there in a negative light (denoting corruption by drink in Semele's [Bacchus's
mother] case, for example).

8. The *Faits des Romains* (The deeds of the Romans), the source of most of the
illustrations used in this book, was an extremely popular text in the Middle Ages that still
exists in several dozen manuscripts. Written by an anonymous northern French clerk in the
early thirteenth century, it was a compilation of translations from Sallust, Suetonius,
Lucan, and Caesar's *De bello gallico,* also known as the *Commentaries.* This last text was also
translated independently into French in later centuries, and its manuscripts also feature
some splendid renditions of the birth of Caesar. Other sources for the *Faits* include Isidore
of Seville's *Etymologies,* glosses and commentaries in manuscripts of Lucan, Flavius
Josephus's *Wars of the Jews,* Saint Augustine, the Bible (to a very small extent), and some
vernacular texts, such as the *Roman de Thèbes* and the *Roman d'Alexandre.*

9. On the uses of medieval illuminations and woodcuts for a reconstruction of the
history of women and children see Alexandre-Bidon and Closson, *L'Enfant,* pp. 7–10.
Their comparison between images and texts makes a convincing case for the realism of
scenes showing births, swaddling, breastfeeding, games, and so on.

10. Previous studies of Caesarean birth almost all have a purely medical perspective and
consider medieval and Renaissance Caesareans only in the context of historical progression (see Young, *Caesarean Section;* Newell, *Caesarean Section;* Levens and Sinz, *Die
künstliche Geburt;* Trolle, *The History of Caesarean Section*). The most comprehensive study
to date is that of Pundel, *L'Histoire.* Although his work is an excellent source book, Pundel
makes no effort to analyze the development of the operation and makes no mention of
the changeover in the performance of Caesarean sections from females to males. He uses
illustrations indiscriminately without any concern for their dates or the texts they come
from. The same defect characterizes a number of medical picture books. Zglinicki, *Die
Geburt* (chap. 5 on Caesarean birth) has many illustrations (one of them [fig. 139] misiden-
tified) but an inadequate text with several errors. Even MacKinney ("Childbirth in the
Middle Ages," p. 234), an expert in the field of medical iconography, makes some incorrect
claims when it comes to Caesareans by stating that midwives were not present in pictures
of Caesarean birth. Other historians (e.g., Hurd-Mead, *A History,* p. 182), ignoring Flutre's
brief 1934 article "La Naissance de César," which clearly shows that the iconographic
tradition of Caesarean birth started in the late thirteenth century, propose that a sixteenth-
century woodcut of Suetonius's *De vita duodecim Caesarum* is the first illustration of a
Caesarean. The same mistake occurs in the catalogue of the British Congress of Obstetrics
and Gynecology (Cambridge, July 1968). Even in a very recent article, the author wrongly
claims that the earliest images of Caesarean birth date from the fifteenth century (Laget,
"La Césarienne," p. 180). The iconography of Caesarean birth, in its development as a *series*
of images as well as in its possible symbolic significance, has never been studied before. The
male incursion into obstetrics has, of course, been explored in the past, but mostly for the
eighteenth and nineteenth centuries. Some excellent material can be found in Donegan,
Women and Men Midwives; Donnison, *Midwives and Medical Men;* Laget, *Naissances;* and
The Male Midwife and the Female Doctor, a collection of primary sources.

1. Caesarean Birth in Medical Thought

1. See the Appendix for medieval thoughts on the etymology of the term "Caesarean
section" and Chapter 4 for legends and miracles relating to Caesarean birth.

2. Gottfried von Strassburg, *Tristan,* trans. A. T. Hatto, p. 63.

3. Rézeau, *Les Prières aux saints*, 2:323–25. All translations are mine, unless otherwise indicated.

4. *De universo* libri XXII (*PL* III, col. 232): "Vipera dicta, quod vi pariat. Nam et venter ejus cum ad partum ingemuerit, catuli non expectantes naturae solutionem, corrosis ejus lateribus, vi erumpunt cum matris interitu. . . . Fertur autem, quod masculus ore inserto viperae semen exspuat, illa autem ex voluptate libidinis in rabiem versa caput matris ore ceptum praecidit. Ita fit, ut parens utraque pereat: masculus dum coit; femina dum parturit" (The viper is called viper because it gives birth by force [*vi*]. When its belly groans with the impending birth, the little ones do not wait for a natural solution but bite through their mother's sides and burst forth, thus causing the mother's destruction. . . . It is said that the male expels the seed while sticking its head into the mouth of the female viper. She is moved by such libidinous and voluptuous frenzy that she bites off the male's head. Thus both parents perish: the male during intercourse, the female while giving birth.) For details on the viper and the Antichrist, see Chapter 4. For a dramatic picture of Saint Margaret emerging from the split belly of the dragon, see B.N. n. acq. fr. 16251 (thirteenth-century; reproduced by Alexandre-Bidon and Closson in *L'Enfant* as plate 4, unfortunately without folio number).

5. Contraception was of course not unknown in this period. It consisted largely of herbal potions, pessaries, and charms. I will discuss this question in Chapter 3 in connection with the activities of medieval midwives. Details can be found in Noonan, *Contraception*. See Laget, *Naissances*, p. 160, for some remarks on the idea that Mary's labor was painless because she had conceived without a man and consequently without pleasure.

6. Bullough, "Medieval Medical and Scientific Views," p. 497.

7. Ibid., p. 499.

8. Davis, "Gender," p. 158.

9. Miles, *Image as Insight*, pp. 89, 93.

10. Noonan, p. 279. Thinkers of the School of Chartres, such as Alanus de Insulis, on the other hand, believed that humans had a duty to procreate. For the School of Chartres, see Wetherbee, *Platonism and Poetry in the Twelfth Century*.

11. The difference between church attitudes and medical ideas is striking. The medical establishment often saw menstruation, intercourse, and pregnancy as beneficial to women. The conflict between religious and medical views did not necessarily have to be resolved, as one can see in the writings of Albertus Magnus. I will consider some of his statements (especially on contraception) in Chapter 3. For details on the differing views of theology and medicine, see Jacquart and Thomasset, *Sexualité*, esp. pp. 265–68. Although the attitudes of the church were on the whole negative, they were much more differentiated than I am able to show here. For an exhaustive treatment of the subject, see Brundage's monumental *Law, Sex, and Christian Society in Medieval Europe*. See also Metz, "Le Statut de la femme en droit canonique médiéval," *Recueil de la Société Jean Bodin* 12 (1962): 59–113; esp. pp. 60–97. Reprinted in Metz, *La Femme et l'enfant*, section 4.

12. Noonan, p. 275.

13. Bullough and Brundage, *Sexual Practices*, p. 206, my emphasis.

14. McNamara, "Chaste Marriage," p. 31.

15. For the problems in getting information on mothers' experiences (if for a somewhat later period), see Wilson, "Participant or Patient?" pp. 129–32. Alexandre-Bidon and Closson provide many pictorial sources for the depiction of medieval mothers and children, but for the medical aspects of childbirth and motherhood their text is not very detailed.

16. Ariès, *L'Enfant et la vie familiale*, p. 134.

17. Ibid., p. 29. See also Laget, *Naissances*, pp. 80–97; she discusses in detail the

paradox of emotional distancing (caused by high infant mortality) and the joyous rituals accompanying the birth of a child.

18. Laget, *Naissances*, p. 134, lists the sometimes insulting names given by men to the women attending a birth.

19. Wilson, p. 141.

20. Ariès, p. 394.

21. *Saints*, p. 47. It seems to me that Weinstein and Bell describe Ariès's position as too extreme, for Ariès states clearly that parental affection existed, that children were not neglected or undervalued. He simply insists on the absence of a "sentiment de l'enfance" (p. 134), i.e., the absence of the consciousness that childhood was a separate stage in life that deserved particular consideration. Children were treated as little adults and had no separate space. One conclusion with regard to Ariès's thesis (drawn neither by Ariès nor by Weinstein and Bell) seems to be that if childhood was undervalued, so was motherhood. In rejecting a separate space for children, society may have effectively denied the special domain of the mother.

22. Hefele and Leclercq, *Histoire*, 5:1575.

23. Shahar, *Die Frau*, p. 105.

24. "Pregnancy," p. 213.

25. Laget, "Childbirth," p. 146.

26. Kealy, *Medieval Medicus*, p. 18.

27. The education and gradual professionalization of midwives will be discussed in Chapter 3.

28. Fasbender, *Geschichte der Geburtshilfe*, p. 15.

29. Soranus of Ephesos, *Soranus' Gynecology*, pp. 69–70.

30. Ibid., p. 71.

31. Ibid., p. 81.

32. Ibid., pp. 97–101.

33. Ibid., pp. 103, 105.

34. Paulus Aegineta, the author of a late antique medical encyclopedia, divides the causes as follows: "Difficult labor arises either from the woman who bears the child, or from the child itself, or from the secundines, or from some external circumstance" (*The Seven Books*, 1:646). Paulus's book is a compilation of ancient authors and he repeats Soranus's advice in many instances. Soranus's remarks are too lengthy to be summarized here. In any case, what interests us primarily is what was retained of Soranus's teachings in the Middle Ages. See the section on Bernard of Gordon (at the beginning of "The Textual Tradition of Caesarean Birth") for details on the reasons for difficult labor.

35. The identity of Trotula (and of the related texts) has been hotly disputed since the sixteenth century. The most recent discussion of the writings and the identity of Trotula can be found in Benton, "Trotula."

36. Rowland, ed., *Medieval Woman's Guide*, p. 42.

37. Soranus, pp. 189–90. See Salvat, "L'Accouchement," p. 98; Paulus Aegineta mentions "powerful shaking" (1:647).

38. Mason-Hohl, *Diseases of Women by Trotula of Salerno*, p. 24.

39. For some recent speculations on what kinds of guidelines were available to midwives as well as on the midwives' possible literacy, see Green, *Toward a History*.

40. For medical education see Talbot, "Medical Education"; McVaugh, "The History of Medicine"; and Siraisi, *Taddeo Alderotti*, chaps. 4 and 5. I will not go into greater detail on Soranus's successors here, since good overviews of medical traditions regarding childbirth, gynecology, and female physiology exist. Old, but still informative is Fasbender. Diepgen, *Frau und Frauenheilkunde*, is excellent, as are Green, *Transmission of Ancient*

Theories, and Jacquart and Thomasset. Salvat is also useful but concentrates mostly on Bartholomeus Anglicus.

41. "Obstetrix autem dicitur mulier que habet artem iuvandi mulierem parientem ut faciliter pariat et infantulus partus tempere periculum non incurat" (Bartholomeus, *De proprietatibus,* fol. 64v). Note that the word used to describe her skills here is *ars* (or "craft" in the Trevisa translation [p. 305]).

42. Bartholomeus, *De proprietatibus,* fol. 64v: "[The midwife] membrorum conforta-tionem delinit membra panniculis involvit. . . . [The wet nurse] fasciis et lintheolis con-stringit membra puerilia et rectificat ea ne aliquam contrabat parvulus curvitatem ipsum deformantem."

43. Salvat, p. 96. Wilson claims (also without any evidence as far as I can ascertain) that, at least for the seventeenth century, swaddling was an important part of the *birth* (not only of infant care): "Indeed there was some tendency to perceive the swaddling-clothes as an integral part of the newborn child. It was these clothes which made the child human" (p. 137). David Hunt suggests that in addition to keeping the baby warm, swaddling was designed to keep infants in a correct posture and to prevent animal-like (and hence undesirable) crawling (*Parents,* pp. 126–30). For Soranus's detailed instructions for swad-dling, see his *Gynecology,* pp. 84–87.

44. See Foucault, *La Naissance de la clinique.*

45. Oppenheim, "A Caesarian Section," p. 292.

46. Forceps are mentioned in the Arabic tradition. See the Cremona translation of Avicenna, 3.21.2.28.

47. See Chapter 2 for a discussion of the illustration and a transcription of the marginal instructions.

48. The text of this law is quoted by Trolle as follows: "Negat lex regia mulierem, quae praegnans mortua sit, humari, antequam partus ei excidatur; qui contra fecerit, spem animantis cum gravida peremisse videtur" (*History of Caesarean Section,* p. 15).

49. Ibid.

50. Pundel, *L'Histoire,* p. 57.

51. Young, *Caesarean Section,* p. 10.

52. *Antiquity of Caesarean Section,* p. 119.

53. Young, p. 10.

54. Ibid.

55. Fasbender, p. 980.

56. Soucek, "An Illustrated Manuscript," p. 111. For details on al-Bīrūnī see the Appen-dix. The illustration is on fol. 16 of manuscript 161 of the Edinburgh University Library. Reproduced in Soucek, fig. 3.

57. In rare cases a physician may have been present at a difficult birth. For an examina-tion of the relevant passages in Arabic writings, see Chapter 3.

58. Ullmann, *Medizin,* pp. 250–51. See Chapter 3 for more details on the role of male physicians or surgeons in gynecological procedures.

59. Salvat, p. 91.

60. See Schipperges's translation (*Heilkunde*) of her medical writings.

61. Cf. MacKinney, *Early Medieval Medicine,* pp. 38–42.

62. Ammundsen, "Medieval Canon Law," p. 28.

63. Pouchelle, "La Prise en charge," p. 251.

64. Ammundsen, p. 31.

65. *Medicine in Medieval England,* p. 55.

66. Ammundsen, p. 41.

67. Wickersheimer, *Commentaires,* p. xlvi. The power struggle between university-

trained physicians, surgeons, barbers, and midwives will be discussed in more detail below and in Chapter 3.

68. *PL* 212, col. 63, no. 6.

69. Hefele and Leclercq, 5:1575.

70. Translated from Hefele, *Conciliengeschichte,* 6:494. Birkelbach, Eifert, and Lueken, "Zur Entwicklung des Hebammenwesens," p. 88, point out that in the Nuremberg midwifery statutes from 1555 the Protestant city council explicitly ordered that unbaptized children should be buried *within* the cemetery walls. Laget shows that the orders of burying unbaptized infants in unconsecrated ground were rarely followed: "car il y a une sorte de répugnance à considérer qu'un enfant réellement né soit écarté de la vie éternelle: elle se traduit par la résistance à enterrer à l'écart des autres les enfants morts à la naissance" (people are repelled by the thought that a child once born should be turned away from the eternal life: this attitude is reflected in the resistance to burying separately those children who had died at birth) (*Naissances,* pp. 312–13).

71. Jacquart, *Le Milieu médical,* p. 50. The idea of using Caesareans in order to attempt baptism of the infant was pushed to extremes by the eighteenth-century inquisitor Cangiamila who, in 1745, published his *Embryologia sacra.* He recommended Caesareans for women who died even in the early stages of pregnancy and called down heavenly wrath on anyone who hesitated to perform this operation. The tenor of his work has been dramatically described by Pundel, pp. 85–91.

72. *Summa theologiae,* 3a.68.11, ed. and trans. James J. Cunningham, 57:116–17. Saint Thomas starts by saying: "Et ideo non debet *homo* occidere matrem. . . ." I chose to translate *homo* as "one" rather than as "man" or "a man," since for the thirteenth century there is no evidence for male participation during the actual birth, not even in the case of a Caesarean. The injunction against killing the mother is thus most likely meant for midwives.

73. Pundel, p. 83.

74. Trolle, p. 21.

75. Rowland, *A Medieval Woman's Guide,* pp. 35–36.

76. Translated from Pouchelle, "La Prise en charge," p. 255. My emphasis.

77. See MacKinney, *Early Medieval Medicine,* for details.

78. Talbot, "Medicine," p. 403.

79. Cf. Imbault-Huart, *La Médecine,* p. 94.

80. "La Prise en charge," p. 258.

81. Talbot, "Medical Education," p. 81.

82. See Pouchelle, "La Prise en charge," p. 260, for some quotes from the text of the *ordonnances* of Charles V specifying what barbers were allowed to do.

83. For details see Riddle, "Theory and Practice."

84. Jacquart, *Le Milieu médical,* p. 200; Pouchelle, "La Prise en charge," p. 259.

85. For a brief but very useful overview, see McVaugh, "History of Medicine," pp. 250–51.

86. Siraisi, p. 109. The list of Lanfranc's topics is not exhaustive, of course. Cf. Lanfranc of Milan, *Science of Surgery.*

87. Thorndike, *A History of Magic and Experimental Science,* 2:479. For the general character of the *Compendia* in this period, see Demaitre, "Scholasticism."

88. See Jacquart and Thomasset, pp. 31 and 48–52, for some examples.

89. Pouchelle, *Corps et chirurgie,* p. 140.

90. Jacquart and Thomasset list some examples on p. 31.

91. There seems to be no unequivocal evidence, however, that this practice was in any way common in the thirteenth century. Cf. Pouchelle, "La Prise en charge," p. 263.

92. For details see Alston, "The Attitude of the Church."

93. Siraisi, p. 110. See also Jacquart and Thomasset, esp. pp. 56–66. They point to the importance of innovative anatomical illustrations (esp. of Guillelmus of Saliceto and Henri de Mondeville, whose work has been studied in detail by Pouchelle in *Corps et chirurgie*). They are cautious to apply the word "progress" to the developments in anatomy, however. Often contradictory findings and texts led to a situation that they describe as somewhat chaotic by the late Middle Ages (p. 49).

94. Siraisi, p. 113.

95. Ibid.,

96. As summarized by Siraisi, ibid., p. 111. For a stunning representation of a medieval dissection, see a fifteenth-century manuscript of Bartholomeus Anglicus's *Des proprietaires des choses* (B.N. f. fr. 218, fol. 218), reproduced in Imbault-Huart, fig. 41 bis. A favorite dissection scene was that of the emperor Nero's mother. Nero, so a medieval legend goes, had his mother dissected so that he could see where he came from. See Chapter 2, nn. 60 and 63, for references to illustrations of this scene.

97. See Pouchelle, "La Prise en charge," p. 268.

98. Ibid., p. 266.

99. See Demaitre, *Doctor Bernard of Gordon,* chap. 1.

100. Ibid., p. 151.

101. "Theory and Practice," p. 120.

102. Ibid., p. 118.

103. Demaitre, *Doctor Bernard of Gordon,* p. 112.

104. Gilbertus's treatise was sometimes called *Laurea anglica.* Together with that work and John of Gaddesdens's later *Rosa anglica,* Bernard's *Practica sive lilium medicinae* (hereafter referred to as *Lilium*) forms the "flower trilogy" of medical treatises. Undoubtedly the *Lilium* is the apex of the series (see Demaitre, *Doctor Bernard of Gordon,* p. 58, and "Scholasticism").

105. Cf. Demaitre, *Doctor Bernard of Gordon,* p. 38.

106. See ibid., esp. chaps. 2 and 4, for a characterization of Bernard's work, and p. 52 n. 83 for the text of Bernard's prologue.

107. Ibid., p. 148.

108. Demaitre is rightly suspicious of "firsts" in medicine (cf. *Doctor Bernard of Gordon,* p. 53), but at the same time he acknowledges Bernard's originality.

109. "Secundo notandum quod foetus potest vivere matre mortua existente saltim per aliquod tempus, nec caret omnino anhelitu, immo foetus attrahit aerem attractum in arteriis matris et potissimem vivit, quando os matricis manet apertum, ideo matre mortua, aliquid artificium debet fieri, ut os matricis stet apertum, et statim venter matricis aperiri foetusque, extrahi et tali artificio, ut dicitur, fuit primus Caesar extractus, indeque ex illo obtinuit nomen" (*Lilium,* fol. 93r). Of the manuscripts I consulted, B.N. f. lat. 15117 repeats the phrase "os matricis" (fol. 78r). B.N. f. lat. 6965, on the other hand, reads "Saltim per aliquod tempus, nec caret omnino anhelitu ymo fetus trahit aerem attractum in arteriis matris et potissime vivit quando *os matris* remanet apertum et ideo matre mortua aliquod artificium debet fieri ut *os matricis* stet apertum etc." (fol. 115v). MS B.N. f. lat. 16189 has first *os matricis* and then *os matris* (fol. 116r). In my opinion, the version of B.N. f. lat. 6995 makes the most sense: first Bernard speaks of the mouth of the mother, then of the mouth of the uterus. The repetition of either *os matris* (although in the early MSS, e.g., B. L. Harley 3698, fol. 95v, or Wellcome Institute Library 130, fol. 137r) or *os matricis* is not as convincing. (For MSS B. L. Harley 3698 and Wellcome 130, I used Demaitre's transcription, which he generously let me see before publication.) Bernard uses the word *artificium* frequently. An *artificium* is always recommended when something natural will not do or cannot be obtained. Cf. Demaitre, *Doctor Bernard of Gordon,* p. 155 n. 5.

110. Soranus also mentions the possibility of an inexperienced physician (p. 182). Bernard omits this reference, a proof that all aspects of obstetrical practice were at that time in the hands of women. See Chapter 3 for a more detailed analysis of possible male involvement in gynecology and obstetrics.

111. These passages of Bernard's work are on fols. 93–94 in the printed edition and on fols. 95 and 96 in B. L. Harley 3698.

112. This passage is followed by the brief remark on Julius Caesar's birth by Caesarean analyzed in the Appendix.

113. Fasbender, p. 98. See Chapter 3 for references to embryotomy and extraction by hooks in Arabic medicine.

114. Nicaise's translation contains several pages of illustrations based on Guy's descriptions; his figures 69 and 70 show razors, one with a mobile blade, the other with a double-edged blade. The latter corresponds to the instruments we can see in a number of manuscript illuminations.

115. "Teneat os mulierum mortue apertum et similiter matrix et hoc ut aer possit ingredi et puer possit evenire. Aperiatur ergo mulier secundum longitudinem ventris cum rasorio in latere sinistro. . . . Ego aliqui feci incisionem a pomo granato usque ad os pectoris cum cautela ne intestinam et puer tangantur. Et per istum modum extraxi puerum; verus primus modus plus placet mihi. Et per hunc modum extractus fuit Julius Cesar: ut scribitur in gestis romanorum." Thus Piero states that of the two ways of doing a Caesarean, i.e., through a lateral or median incision, he prefers the first.

116. "Nam pro pauperculis non multum laborat medicus" (cited by Fasbender, p. 104).

117. Diepgen, p. 201.

118. German text in Ketsch, *Frauen im Mittelalter,* 1:286.

119. This observation will be confirmed in the discussion of the statutes of midwives in Chapter 3.

120. Translated from the edition by M. Schleissner, lines 1676–78.

121. See Fasbender, p. 134, and Guillemeau's letter to Rousset discussed below.

122. *Oeuvres complètes,* vol. 2, chap. 38.

123. Ibid., 2:717.

124. Ibid., 2:718.

125. For some observations on the controversy (and especially the anti-Caesarean school of Citoyen Sacombe) in the late eighteenth century, see Laget, *Childbirth,* pp. 171–72. Apropos of Caesarean section, she concludes that the criteria of what constitutes death were not fully defined and that "surgical procedures [i.e., Caesarean sections] performed on living but exhausted, half-conscious, or crazed women, affected those who witnessed them as a scandalous, barbaric, and traumatic experience" (p. 171).

126. Young, *Caesarean Section,* p. 25.

127. Ibid.

128. Rousset, *Traitté,* p. 137.

129. Rousset never made good on this promise. His treatise was translated into Latin by Caspar Bauhin in 1582. It was printed in many editions.

130. Rousset, pp. 7, 8.

131. Ibid., p. 11.

132. Ibid., p. 12.

133. Ibid., pp. 16, 18, 19, 21.

134. Ibid., pp. 25, 29.

135. Ibid., p. 26.

136. The practice of suturing the uterus after a Caesarean was introduced by Lebas in 1769. The technique became widely known only in 1882 when Max Sänger published his

Leipzig dissertation, "Der Kaiserschnitt bei Uterusfibromen nebst vergleichender Methodik der sectio caesarea und der Porro-Operation."

137. Cited by Pundel, p. III.

138. Rousset, p. 125.

139. Young, p. 23; Pundel, pp. 117–19.

140. The texts chronicling the controversy over Caesareans on living women were available to me on a microfilm from the John Rylands Library at the University of Manchester. They are bound in one volume. They are (1) François Rousset, *Dialogus apologeticus pro Caesareo partu cuiusdam pseudoprotei dicteria* (Paris: Denys Duval, 1590); (2) Jacques Marchant, *In Fr. Rosseti Apologiam, Declamatio* (Paris: Nicolaus Delouvain, 1598); (3) Jacques Guillemeau, *Francisco Rosseto* (inserted in the Marchant text just cited, pp. 37–44); (4) Jacques Marchant, *In Fr. Rosseti librum de Caesareo partu. Carmen* (texts [2]–[4] are paginated continuously); (5) Jacques Marchant, *Declamatio III in Fr. Rosseti* (there seems to be no *Declamatio II* unless the poem [4] is counted); (6) Jacques Marchant, *Carmen;* (7) François Rousset, *Responsio ad Jacobi Marchant Declamationem* (Paris, n.d.). This last part is in manuscript form in the Manchester copy. I will refer to the texts by the number I assigned them in this note.

141. (1), p. 5, 6, 8, 14, 24–31, 35, 37.

142. (2), p. 14.

143. (2), pp. 18, 19.

144. (3), pp. 39, 40, 42, 44.

145. (5), pp. 16, 29, 30.

146. (6), p. 2.

147. Book 2, chap. 28. For a long time this text had been assigned to the seventeenth century (Fasbender, p. 135). Some of the passages of *La commare* on Caesarean section were translated into Spanish in 1966 by Sanchez Arcas, "Contribución."

148. *La commare,* book 2, pp. 216, 208, 212 (quotations); 207, 212.

149. P. 4.

2. Caesarean Birth in the Artistic Imagination

1. Cf., e.g., Meier and Ruberg, *Text und Bild; Texte et image;* Curschmann, "Hören"; Miles, *Image as Insight.* Somewhat older but also important is Pickering, *Literatur und darstellende Kunst.*

2. A very useful collection of medieval sources was published by Ketsch in *Frauen im Mittelalter,* vol. 1. See also Fox, *The Medieval Woman;* Hanawalt, *Women and Work.*

3. The term "profession" is of course anachronistic in the context of medieval midwifery. I use it here with the understanding that early midwifery exhibited few of the traits one associates with the modern notion of "professionalism."

4. The images of Caesarean birth are particularly valuable because those of normal childbirth featured no men and thus offer no possibility of comparison.

5. Wilson highlights the distinction between the different female participants in a birth scene: "The mother and the midwife were formally distinct; even though they were both women, this does not imply that their viewpoints were identical; and the fact that we tend to assume a shared 'women's view' may be a product of our late twentieth century feminism" ("Participant or Patient?", p. 130). See also n. 78 in this context.

6. Jacobsen, "Pregnancy," p. 93. These categories are meant to refer to the content of the sources, not their "originator or originatrix" (ibid.). This division may be applicable to certain types of texts, such as the ones Jacobsen is analyzing—ballads composed for special occasions in which only women were participating. Jacobsen's categories are more difficult

to apply to illustrations, but they should be taken into account nonetheless. With regard to childbirth, Jacobsen states, "the sources categorized as women's sources describe the process of pregnancy and childbirth from women's point of view and illuminate the perception women had of their biological functions, whereas men's sources deal with men's views or perceptions of reproduction. Common sources are those which provide a perspective on the topic that is gender-neutral" (p. 93). In an ideal world we would be able to know which type of source we are dealing with in any given case. As it is, we are—especially for the medieval period—often groping in the dark.

7. Labarge, *A Small Sound,* p. 230.

8. Ibid., p. 231.

9. Farquhar and Hindman, *Pen to Press,* p. 67.

10. See the annotated list of illustrations for any known information on painters.

11. P. 33.

12. Pp. 89, 93.

13. *The Lady and the Virgin,* chap. 3.

14. Herrlinger, *Geschichte der medizinischen Abbildung,* vol. 1, p. 9; examples of the five-picture cycle and the sixth picture, pp. 10–14.

15. For examples see Jones, *Medieval Medical Miniatures,* fig. 29, and Imbault-Huart, *Médecine médiévale,* plates 15–18.

16. A bloodletting man can be seen in Jones, figs. 54 and 55; Imbault-Huart, plate 46. A cautery man appears in Jones, fig. 43. Wound men are depicted in Jones, figs. 2 and 51. Other types of medical illustrations, not central to our interests here, are listed in MacKinney, *Medical Illustrations.* They include representations of hospitals and clinics; diagnosis and prognosis (by uroscopy, pulse reading, and astrology); pharmacy; external and internal medication; orthopedics; dentistry; bathing; veterinary medicine.

17. A page of this manuscript is reproduced in Jones, plate 9. See also Herrlinger, vol. 1, plate 12.

18. This is MS Ashmole 399. No text is attached to these illustrations and they have given rise to a number of speculations as to their significance. For details see MacKinney, "A Thirteenth-Century Medical Case History."

19. Singer, "Thirteenth-Century Miniatures," p. 74. MacKinney mentions a possible "rival": a fourth-century catacomb mural ("Childbirth," p. 254).

20. According to Singer, "Thirteenth-Century Miniatures."

21. See Grape-Albers, p. 86.

22. The following is a summary of Sudhoff's *Beiträge zur Geschichte der Chirurgie* 10 (1914), pp. 69–70.

23. MacKinney, *Medical Illustrations,* p. 86.

24. Often reproduced, e.g., in Lehmann, *Die Geburt in der Kunst,* p. 59; Grape-Albers, *Spätantike Bilder,* p. 81. A facsimile edition of this codex was edited by C. H. Talbot and F. Unterkircher as *Medica antiqua.* A similar illustration can be found in Florence, Biblioteca Laurenziana, MS Plut. 73, 16, fol. 127v. Cf. MacKinney, *Medical Illustrations,* p. 81.

25. Grape-Albers, p. 3.

26. It also was supposed to have many other properties related to contraceptives and aphrodisiacs (cf. Noonan, *Contraception,* pp. 203–18).

27. Cf. Soranus, *Gynecology,* pp. 73–74.

28. Sudhoff, *Beiträge,* 10:3.

29. Vol. 1, p. 52.

30. The illustration from al-Bīrūnī's *Chronicle of Ancient Nations* mentioned in Chapter 1 (Soucek, "Illustrated Manuscripts," fig. 3) was not made for a medical text, but it certainly shows that Arabic illustrators were capable of showing a medical procedure.

31. Illustration in Speert, *Iconographia,* p. 387.

32. Lehmann, p. 46.

33. This is MS 3714 of the Royal Library at Brussels. Cf. Herrlinger, vol. 1, p. 22. Temkin, in his translation of Soranus's *Gynecology,* reproduces two pages of this manuscript: fig. 1 shows the horned uterus; fig. 2, positions of the fetus.

34. Imbault-Huart, illus. 52, pp. 122–23.

35. Lehmann, figs. 39 and 40.

36. Lehmann, fig. 38.

37. Salomon, *Opicinus de Canistris,* vol. 2, p. 320.

38. See Rowland, *A Medieval Woman's Guide,* pp. 124–33; Pansier, "Un Manuel"; Roesslin; Imbault-Huart, illus. 53 (B.N. lat. 7056), dated about the end of the thirteenth or beginning of the fourteenth century.

39. Lehmann, pp. 17ff.

40. Ibid.

41. Grape-Albers, illus. 187 (B.N. n. acq. lat. 2334, fol. 22v). This picture is in the collection of Ektachromes of the Bibliothèque Nationale. The illustration in the *Wenzelsbibel* is reproduced in Harksen, *Die Frau,* p. 94. It shows a fully dressed woman in a squatting position; her hands are folded. A midwife is receiving a baby from between the woman's legs. Unfortunately Harksen does not indicate the folio number for this illustration or which biblical birth it represents.

42. This "propping up" is an iconographic element called "Stützmotiv" by Grape-Albers. The manuscript in question is Leipzig Cod. 417, fol. 6v. The illustration is number 189 in Grape-Albers.

43. No. 1923.15 in the Fogg Art Museum in Cambridge, Mass.

44. Müllerheim, *Die Wochenstube in der Kunst;* the exceptions are illustrations from the treatise by Roesslin mentioned in Chapter 1. (There are also illustrations in Jacob Rueff's *De conceptu et generatione hominis* [Zürich, 1554].)

45. See Müllerheim, fig. 57. Another striking example is a painting from an altar in Tirol (ca. 1372) that shows the Virgin nude to the waist (Harksen, plate 94).

46. Cf. Cornell, *Iconography of the Nativity,* chap. 1.

47. P. 108. Examples can be found in Jones (front of the dust jacket shows British Library, Royal MS 15 E II, fol. 165); Imbault-Huart, illus. 26 (B.N. fr. 22532), 27 (B.N. fr. 22531), and 42 (B.N. fr. 218).

48. P. 125.

49. Glasgow, University of Glasgow MS Hunter 112 (fourteenth–fifteenth century). The illumination in question is mistakenly listed by MacKinney as a Caesarean section (*Medical Illustrations,* p. 128, no. 66.5).

50. This is MS B.N. f. fr. 2030. For an excellent study of Henri de Mondeville, see Pouchelle, *Corps et chirurgie.*

51. Such as the head operation on fol. 2, reproduced in Jones, plate 9. (The same illustration on the back of the dust jacket is identified as being on fol. 6 instead of fol. 2.)

52. Jones, p. 28. The manuscript is Bodleian Library, Additional MS 36617, fol. 28v. Reproduced in Jones, fig. 7. For the correct representation of the speculum, see the Leclerc translation of Abulcasis, fig. 103.

53. In addition to such schematic illustrations as zodiac women or "disease women," Jones, plate 2, shows a woman with the names of internal organs and diseases written over the figure; "high on her left side is a flask-shaped embryo" (p. 48; from the Wellcome Apocalypse, MS 49, fol. 38).

54. Jones, p. 34, fig. 9.

55. Probably not a "wife," as Labarge, p. 170, suggests. This illustration is from J. du Ries's *Quart volume d' histoire scolastique,* B.L., Royal 15 MS D I, fol. 18. It is reproduced in Ketsch vol. 1, illus. 409; Fox (page for September 13–18); and Labarge, illus. 40.

56. This picture comes from MS 2644, fol. 53v, of the National Library in Vienna. It is reproduced in Fox (December 19–24); Ketsch, plate 443; Cogliati Arano, *Tacuinum sanitatis* (in the English translation by Ratti and Westbrook), plate 41.

57. Jones, fig. 56.

58. The Index of Christian Art at Princeton University has hundreds of entries for the depiction of midwives. They appear in manuscript illuminations, on stained-glass windows and ivory, on sculptures, frescoes, and metalwork. Most of these listings are for the Nativity, the birth of Saint John or Mary or other biblical figures.

59. P. 144.

60. Holländer studied only one image, a woodcut from a 1506 Venetian edition of Suetonius's *De vita duodecim Caesarum* (reproduced in Holländer, fig. 85; Pundel, *L'Histoire*, fig. 7; Huard and Grmek, *Mille ans de Chirurgie*, fig. 154; and elsewhere). This seems to be the most frequently reproduced representation of a Caesearean section. Hurd-Mead, *A History*, p. 182, seriously suggests that this sixteenth-century illustration is the first representation of a Caesarean section. In general, Hurd-Mead's illustrations are unreliable; in several cases they are approximate sketches from manuscripts. The most glaring error is the illustration on p. 216, which supposedly shows two female surgeons. It is actually a picture from Roland of Parma's *Chirurgia* (MS Rome Biblioteca Casanatense 1382) showing two male surgeons wearing surgical caps. I thank one of the readers for Cornell University Press for supplying this reference. The usefulness of illustrations for medical history is often undercut by historians of medicine themselves who use illustrations without paying much attention to the texts they come from or to the dates or provenances of the manuscripts. Thus Lehmann gives no clues as to which manuscripts he used; Speert's picture credits are just as deficient. One also has to beware of pressing one's own interpretation upon a given illustration. Thus Carstensen, Schadewaldt, and Vogt commit a major gaffe in their *Chirurgie in der Kunst* when they reflect on the supposed bloody realism of what they believe is a Caesarean birth (illus. 5, p. 18). The fact that there is no baby to be seen should have given them pause: the manuscript reveals that the scene shows the dissection of Nero's mother, performed by a low surgeon and watched anxiously by a bearded Nero. Even such a thorough study as Pundel's uses illuminations from the fourteenth, fifteenth, and sixteenth centuries without discriminating between them.

61. Quoted in the Appendix.

62. For the notion of "conceptualizer," see Brenk, "Le Texte et l'image."

63. A good example of this type of intestine can be seen in a fifteenth-century manuscript of a translation of Boccaccio's *De casibus* (Paris, Bibliothèque de l'Arsenal, MS fr. 5193, fol. 290v). The scene is the same as the one mentioned above: Nero is watching the dissection of his mother. Another splendid example from ca. 1500 is on fol. 59 of Harley MS 4425 of the British Library (reproduced in Jones, plate 3). Again a short-robed surgeon is performing the autopsy while Nero, dressed as a Roman emperor, looks on. The intestines in all these representations are rolled up in a spiral shape.

64. Wiesner, "Early Modern Midwifery," p. 97.

65. These figures apply to late medieval Nuremberg and have been worked out by Wiesner (p. 97). See Chapters 1 and 3 for details of midwives' ordinances specifying the rules they had to follow for Caesarean sections.

66. Keupper Valle, in her survey of Caesareans performed in Alta California between 1769 and 1833, cites two days as the longest survival period of a newborn delivered by Caesarean. The cases of supposedly successful Caesareans discussed in Chapter 1 were clearly the exception.

67. For details see Birkelbach, Eifert, and Lueken, "Zur Entwicklung des Hebammenwesens"; Wiesner; and Chapter 3.

68. The curtain motif connects figures 6, 7, and 8. Figure 8, dated by Flutre in *Les*

Manuscrits as late thirteenth century, shows many characteristics that point to a later date, probably the second quarter of the fourteenth century. (I thank Adelaide Bennett of the Index of Christian Art at Princeton University for her advice on the dating of these miniatures.)

69. Despite repeated efforts (over several years) I have not been able to obtain reproductions of the illuminations in manuscripts 726 and 770 from the Musée Condé in Chantilly.

70. The caption of figure 9 as it is reproduced in Fox (illustration for week of July 7) is "Woman surgeon performing Caesarean section."

71. On the existence of the "surgeoness," see Chapter 3.

72. Weindler, "Der Kaiserschnitt," figs. 7 and 8. Since many of the manuscripts of the *Faits des Romains* also contain a universal chronicle called the *Histoire ancienne jusqu'à César* (which starts with the creation of the world), the "birth" of Eve was often shown in the same manuscript as Caesar's birth. An illuminator thus may have been tempted to use an identical pattern for the two births.

73. One of the early (fourteenth-century) examples falls into neither category. In the only Italian example (fig. 11; Venetian according to Wyss, *Die Caesarteppiche,* p. 50), from the Biblioteca San Marco in Venice, a male surgeon just delivered the child with the help of a midwife and a female attendant. In Italy, the evolution of the medical profession was different from that in France and consequently the presence of a male surgeon as early as the fourteenth century is not too surprising.

74. *Medieval Medicus,* p. 18.

75. For the former we have one example: fig. 18; for the latter, two examples: fig. 15 and fig. 16. For details on the texts see Flutre, *"Li Faits des Romains."*

76. The crane was thought to be a symbol of prudence and vigilance, wisdom and foresight. For the full symbolism of the crane, see Rowland, *Birds with Human Souls,* pp. 31–35.

77. For the sometimes very high salaries of medieval surgeons, see Hammond, "Incomes."

78. This picture provides an excellent caveat against stereotypical thinking. Do women have a gentler nature just because they are women? John Benton, "Trotula," p. 47, observes with regard to the three treatises (wrongly) attributed to Trotula for many centuries: "Though they bear the name of a female author, I must say that throughout these three treatises I see no evidence of the 'gentle hand of a woman' or that the medicine prescribed, as another writer has said, is 'remarkable for its humanity.'" As it turns out, the three treatises in question were written by men, so that "the gentle hand of a woman," apparently detected by Hurd-Mead (in "Trotula," *Isis* 14 [1930], pp. 364–65) is no more than a fiction produced by wishful and stereotypical thinking.

79. Cf. Feis, "Bericht aus dem Jahre 1411."

80. Even such skilled artists as Dürer and Leonardo da Vinci made such "mistakes." As Gombrich points out in *Art and Illusion:* "Apparently not even Dürer knew what 'eyes really look like.' This should not give us cause for surprise, for the greatest of all the visual explorers, Leonardo himself, has been shown to have made mistakes in his anatomical drawings. Apparently he drew features of the human heart which Galen made him expect but which he cannot have seen" (pp. 82–83). As shown in the previous chapter, human dissection did not necessarily lead to the correction of some of the ancient authorities' misconceptions.

81. Cf. Gold, p. 61.

82. Figure 21, from the Wellcome Apocalypse (Wellcome Library MS 49) is the only medical illustration of the operation I could find. The other illustration (reproduced in Pundel, fig. 19) is from a model book (fig. 197* d 2 of the Department of Prints and

Engravings of the British Library) of medical scenes but does not illustrate a medical text. It shows the technique of holding open the mother's mouth (fol. 16). Another scene from the same book can be seen in Jones, fig. 52; it shows an operation for scrotal hernia. Thus, for Caesareans, the same paradox that I described for the iconography of childbirth in general holds true: they were represented frequently and lavishly in historical manuscripts, but rarely in medical manuscripts. The figure of Julius Caesar, who had captured the medieval imagination, clearly inspired illustrators much more than the operation as such, associated as it was with death.

3. The Marginalization of Women in Obstetrics

1. Cf. Donegan, *Women and Men Midwives;* Donnison, *Midwives and Medical Men;* Ehrenreich and English, *Witches, Midwives, and Nurses.* Men may have been present earlier at royal births, as noted in Chapter 1.

2. P. 4.

3. Rosenberg, "The Medical Profession," p. 24.

4. Ibid., p. 25.

5. For an astute evaluation of this type of "tunnel history" for the history of obstetrics, see Wilson, "Participant or Patient?" pp. 129–30.

6. Ehrenreich and English, p. 13.

7. *The Medical Man,* p. 58.

8. Barstow, from the State University of New York, College at Old Westbury, has analyzed the male bias in the historiography of witchcraft in her paper "On Studying Witchcraft." I thank her for letting me see this paper in manuscript form. Biased scholarship on midwives is not a male prerogative, however. In *Midwives in History and Society,* Jean Towler and Joan Bramall seem to be unaware of the ideological biases present in the stories from the *Malleus maleficarum.* In fact, they seem to "buy" the evidence of treatises on witchcraft when they say, "There is evidence that witches, having summoned up the devil and other evil spirits, indulged in incestuous orgies. . . . If the witches were not midwives themselves, this practice [baking the ashes of newborn babies] would have required collusion (perhaps under threat) with the midwives" (p. 37). I have the impression that Towler and Bramall, in writing a history of midwives, want to exonerate midwives at the expense of "witches."

9. *World of the Witches,* p. 256.

10. *The Midwife and the Witch,* p. 139.

11. One example that can stand for many is Gubalke, *Die Hebamme,* p. 64.

12. Cited in Benedek, "The Changing Relationship," p. 552. For details of the trial, see Kibre, "The Faculty of Medicine."

13. Cf. Rosenthal, "Zur geburtshilflich-gynäkologischen Betätigung des Mannes," p. 128.

14. Soranus, *Gynecology,* pp. 182, 184, 192.

15. For details, see Rosenthal, pp. 133–37, and Ullmann, *Medizin in Islam,* pp. 250–51.

16. Abulcasis, *Chirurgie,* p. 182.

17. The translation from the Arabic was supplied by George Saliba from Columbia University. The grammatical forms of the address to the reader indicate that Rhazes is speaking to a man all along. The Latin passage in the *Continens* reads: "Quod si opus fuerit quod fiat operatio cum ferro sedeat mulier super scamnum que admodum sedere debet penes partu [i.e., the birth stool]: et post dorsum retrorsum debet extrahere alius cui adhereat: deinde *medicus* sedeat super genu dextrum ut sequens possit quod ad velle erit et aperienda enim vulva cum instrumentu tortuli vel torculi volventis cum inde aperiatur os

matricis et egrediatur secundina" (vol. 1, fol. 196r b). The Arabic text, which is arranged somewhat differently from the Latin, has this passage on p. 100 in part 9. The Arabic *mu'ālij* does not exactly correspond to Latin *medicus*. It is a very general term for a person involved in medical activities. But, and this is the important point, it always refers to a man.

18. *Kitāb al-Ḥāwī fī al-Ṭibb,* pt. 9, p. 137.

19. P. 174.

20. This passage is in *Canon,* 3.21.2.28. (there are no page or folio numbers in the edition I used). This chapter is famous for its mention of forceps (*forcipes*), which the midwife should use to extract the child. If the child cannot be extracted this way, the midwife should remove the child "by incision" (with hooks) and on the whole proceed as if the child were dead ("regimine fetus mortui").

21. Siraisi, *Taddeo Alderotti,* p. 280, n. 42.

22. Ibid., p. 279.

23. Cited in Rosenthal, p. 39.

24. Lemay, "Anthonius Guainerius and Medieval Gynecology," p. 322.

25. This is miracle number 8 in the collection *Vierge et merveille. Les miracles de Notre-Dame narratifs au moyen âge.*

26. Bullough, *The Development of Medicine,* pp. 52 and 69.

27. For details see ibid.

28. Wickersheimer, *Commentaires,* p. lxxvi.

29. Bullough, *The Development of Medicine,* p. 85; Wickersheimer, *Commentaires,* p. lxxvii.

30. The details of this complicated fight can be found in Wickersheimer, *Commentaires.* See also Pouchelle, "La Prise en charge," pp. 258ff.

31. Bullough, *The Development of Medicine,* p. 86.

32. P. lxxxiv.

33. Feis, "Bericht aus dem Jahre 1411," p. 340.

34. Hughes, *Women Healers,* p. 86.

35. Jacquart, *Le Milieu médical,* p. 47.

36. This information is based on ibid., pp. 48–53. See also Wickersheimer's *Dictionnaire* and Jacquart's *Supplément au Dictionnaire.*

37. *Le Milieu médical,* p. 51.

38. Lipinska, *Histoire des femmes médecins,* p. 182.

39. Hurd-Mead, *A History,* p. 370.

40. Jacquart, *Le Milieu médical,* p. 52.

41. Ibid.

42. Cited by Hurd-Mead, p. 215.

43. Jacquart, *Le Milieu médical,* p. 79. For some information on the early Middle Ages, see MacKinney, *Early Medieval Medicine.* On the role of surgery in the education of physicians at Montpellier, see Demaitre, *Doctor Bernard of Gordon.*

44. Jones, *Medieval Medical Miniatures,* p. 123.

45. Ibid., fig. 56.

46. Hughes, p. 89.

47. Ibid.

48. Kibre, p. 12.

49. See ibid. and Bullough, *The Development of Medicine,* for details.

50. Cited by Nicaise in his introduction to Guy de Chauliac, p. lxiv.

51. The following is a summary of chaps. 1 and 2 of book 1 of Soranus's *Gynecology,* pp. 5–7.

52. Fasbender, *Geschichte der Geburtshilfe,* p. 78.

53. Ibid., p. 79.

54. See Benton, "Trotula," for the definitive word on Trotula and other women practitioners in Salerno.

55. On questions of the learning of midwives, gynecological texts, and their audiences, see Green, "Toward a History."

56. See Benton; Green, *The Transmission of Ancient Theories*. For one of the English translations, see Rowland, *A Medieval Woman's Guide*.

57. For details on this text, see Lemay.

58. For the idea of the "sharing of literacy" on the communal level, see Stock, *Implications of Literacy*.

59. "Early Modern Midwifery," p. 107.

60. For the texts of the relevant canons of several church councils, see Chapter 1.

61. Wiesner, p. 96.

62. A portion of this text is printed (in a modernized form) in Ketsch, *Frauen im Mittelalter*, 1:280–82. In addition to Wiesner, see Birkelbach, Eifert, and Lueken, "Zur Entwicklung des Hebammenwesens," for a study of these regulations.

63. The ordinance is not quite clear on the reasons for such drastic measures. Possibly the text refers to the burial of an unbaptized infant in consecrated ground.

64. The German term is *unterwinden*, a curious but picturesque term, literally meaning "to twist under."

65. Text in Ketsch, 1:282–84.

66. See Birkelbach, Eifert, and Lueken, p. 91. See also below.

67. P. 99.

68. Petrelli, "The Regulation of French Midwifery," p. 277. For the seventeenth and eighteenth centuries, see Gélis, "La Formation des accoucheurs et des sages-femmes."

69. P. 82.

70. Cash, "The Birth of Tristram Shandy," p. 141. See also Wilson: "To call the surgeon was to abandon the ceremony [of childbirth], to surrender hope for the life of the child, and to subject the mother to a terrifying operation. Consequently women put off this step until the last possible minute" (p. 137).

71. Cf. the comments of Eccles: "Obstetrics did of course change profoundly between the sixteenth and the eighteenth centuries, two of the most obvious changes being the invention of the obstetric forceps, and the irruption of men into midwifery practice. It is not so certain that the result was altogether an improvement. The ignorant, harsh and vulgar midwife who first appeared as a verbal cartoon figure in this period was sometimes replaced by the licentious, instrument-happy, self-serving man-midwife who also appeared as a cartoon figure a little later" (*Obstetrics and Gynaecology in Tudor and Stuart England*, p. 87). See also Laget's revealing remarks on the subject (*Naissances*, pp. 208–13).

72. Barstow, p. 7, n. 1.

73. Kieckhefer, *European Witch Trials*, p. 11.

74. The *Malleus*, belonging as it does to the learned tradition, stresses demonic possession as the origin of most witchcraft practices. That most frequently this possession was thought of as sexual possession fits well into the obsessive pattern of sadism and voyeurism that characterizes the *Malleus* and other later treatises. For a good analysis of the logical flaws and absurd reasoning in the *Malleus*, see Anglo, "Evident Authority and Authoritative Evidence: The *Malleus maleficarum*." The distinction between the learned and popular (or clerical and secular) traditions is not absolute, of course. *Maleficia* also appeared in learned (medical) texts.

75. Thomas, *Religion and the Decline of Magic*; Macfarlane, *Witchcraft in Tudor and Stuart England*.

76. Monter, *Witchcraft in France and Switzerland*, pp. 193–94.

77. Midelfort, *Witch Hunting in Southwestern Germany*, p. 12.

78. Kieckhefer, p. 12.

79. Cf. Nelson, "Why Witches Were Women," and Russell, *Witchcraft in the Middle Ages.*

80. Monter, p. 141.

81. Midelfort, p. 184.

82. Monter, p. 124.

83. See Bullough, "Medieval Medical and Scientific Views of Women." In a remarkable article, Michèle Ouerd examines the similarity between the vocabulary used in the witch trials and that used by nineteenth-century medical writers on female hysteria. The misogynistic imagery, centering as it does on the concept of "possession," is almost identical in both areas.

84. Midelfort, p. 13.

85. Trans. Montague Summers, p. 41. All references will be to this translation. There is also a good French translation of the *Malleus* by Amand Danet, with a lengthy and very informative introduction.

86. Institoris and Sprenger, pt. 2, p. 118.

87. Story cited by Towler and Bramall, pp. 35–36 (Institoris and Sprenger, chap. 13). Towler's and Bramall's comments to this story are limited to "Much of this tale seems in present times rather far-fetched but at the time of telling would, in almost every detail, be believed" (p. 36). See n. 8 to this chapter for an evaluation of Towler's and Bramall's approach.

88. Birkelbach, Eifert, and Lueken, p. 91.

89. A radical thesis on the destruction of the wise women of the Middle Ages was published in Germany in 1985 by Heinsohn and Steiger, *Vernichtung der weisen Frauen.* The authors contend that the witch-hunts as a whole must be seen as a campaign (engineered from "above") against contraception. Since in the fourteenth century Europe lost a large part of its population, they argue, the work force was critically diminished. In order to spur population growth a policy was adopted by the ruling classes whose aim it was to eliminate all knowledge that could curb the birth rate. Heinsohn's and Steiger's arguments are intriguing, but their documentation is not quite convincing. Evidence for a coherent "policy" of encouraged population growth is either nonexistent or too late to buttress their argument. Demographic studies do not support their arguments either. A dramatic increase in the European population is not visible until the eighteenth century (Nelson, p. 346). Also, the authors do not take into account the important regional variations in the witch-hunts. In England, for example, the sexual element was much less important than in Germany. Very little remains of their thesis after careful examination, but nonetheless the study has some merits: it confirms that one of the central concerns, if not the only one, of the witch-hunts was the elimination of knowledge proper to the "wise women." See also Horsley and Horsley, "On the Trail of the Witches," p. 26 n. 31, for a critique of a 1982 article by Heinsohn and Steiger that presented the same theses as their later book.

90. For a recent comprehensive study, see Brundage, *Law, Sex and Christian Society.*

91. Noonan, *Contraception,* pp. 44, 48, 100, 129.

92. For the text see *Corpus scriptorum ecclesiasticorum latinorum,* vol. 42 (Vienna, 1902), pp. 229–30.

93. See Jacquart and Thomasset, *Sexualité,* chap. 3, esp. pp. 119–30, for a judicious treatment of medical and theological views on contraception.

94. Hansen, *Zauberwahn,* p. 359.

95. For an example see Institoris and Sprenger, p. 122.

96. Ibid., p. 119.

97. Contraception has to be distinguished from sterility, which was undesirable in women. Witches were also reputed for "withering the fruit" of pregnant women and

keeping them from becoming pregnant again. These matters are quite different from desired contraception, which would allow women some control over their bodies.

98. Payer, *Sex and the Penitentials,* p. 34.

99. Noonan, p. 207.

100. Ibid., p. 205.

101. Cf. Jacquart and Thomasset, pp. 265–68.

102. Noonan, p. 230.

103. Ibid., p. 365.

104. The authors never address the problem of the proportion between the number of people killed in the witch-hunts and the number of births that took place because of the elimination of contraception and abortion.

105. Le Maistre, *Quaestiones morales,* vol. 2, fol. 48v (quoted by Noonan, p. 307).

106. See his *Quellen,* pp. 416–44. The section is entitled "Die Zuspitzung des Hexen-wahns auf das weibliche Geschlecht" (The intensification of the witchcraft mania directed against the female sex).

107. Peters, *The Magician, the Witch, and the Law,* p. 170. One should not forget that similar crimes of infanticide and intercourse with the devil were attributed to Jews and heretics in the Middle Ages. For details see Moore, *The Formation of a Persecuting Society,* pp. 36–37, 64.

108. Institoris and Sprenger, p. 66.

109. *An Examen of Witches,* p. 88.

110. Hansen, *Quellen,* p. 542. For medieval views on masturbation and the nature of menstrual blood, see Jacquart and Thomasset, chaps. 2 and 4.

111. Trexler, "Infanticide in Florence," p. 101.

112. Described in detail by Barstow, in an as yet unpublished paper that will be part of her forthcoming study on witchcraft.

113. Brissaud, p. 246.

114. Ibid., pp. 250–53.

115. Bergues, "Prévention des naissances," p. 197.

116. P. 107. The connection between accusations of witchcraft and possibly real crimes has been explored by Midelfort: "It is sometimes asserted that witchcraft was a *Modev-erbrechen,* a fashionable crime under which many old-fashioned, genuine crimes were subsumed. There can be no doubt that in the many small, isolated witchcraft trials that went on throughout the sixteenth and seventeenth centuries, many crimes like fornication, abortion, infanticide, and poisoning were connected to witchcraft. It is another matter, however, to assert that those caught up in severe witch panics were real criminals. One would then be faced with explaining a sudden crime wave of enormous proportions" (p. 187).

117. P. 187.

118. See n. 50.

119. Becker et al., *Aus der Zeit der Verzweiflung,* p. 330.

120. Hansen, *Quellen,* p. 542.

121. Heinsohn and Steiger, p. 150.

122. This is why there was firm belief in miracles relating to the resurrection of unbaptized newborns. A split-second resurrection would suffice to baptize the infant. The mother's need for the assurance of her child's salvation accounts for the large number of miracles related to this problem. Of the fifty-six miracles attributed to the fifteenth-century saint Philippe Chantemilan, for example, almost twenty involved the momentary re-suscitation of newborns (Paravy, "L'Angoisse collective," p. 92). On the question of the midwives' dispensing of baptism, see also Laget, *Naissances,* pp. 307–12.

123. Wiesner, p. 107.

124. Heinsohn and Steiger, p. 132.

125. See Birkelbach, Eifert, and Lueken, pp. 85ff., for details.

126. According to ibid., p. 86.

127. See Laget, *Naissances,* pp. 208ff. She shows that, at least in theory, in the seventeenth and eighteenth centuries male obstetrical practice was equated with "scientific" and with the use of instruments.

128. See Katharine Park, *Doctors and Medicine in Early Renaissance Florence,* for the effects of the Great Plague on the medical profession. Midelfort, p. 12, develops the idea of the scapegoat in relation to the Great Plague.

129. That does not mean that the two movements are causally related. Although they do overlap in several areas, one is not the consequence of the other.

4. Saintly and Satanic Obstetricians

1. The term *himmlischer Gynaekologe* is used by Ernst Richter in "Die Opferung," the article from which much of the material on this special cult is drawn.

2. The traditional iconography of Saint Roch shows him standing holding a pilgrim's staff and wearing a pilgrim's hat (often with the emblem of Compostella, a scallop shell). At his feet sit a dog and/or an angel. The dog often holds a piece of bread in his mouth: an offering to the shunned sufferer of the plague. Saint Roch's right hand normally points to his thigh wound, the sign of his suffering.

3. Richter, p. 77.

4. Ibid., p. 82.

5. For the various beliefs and superstitions that surrounded childbirth, see Sanchez Arcas, "Creencias, supersticiónes, y mitos." On saints in charge of childbirth, see Pachinger, *Die Mutterschaft,* pp. 185ff. The most curious "saint" mentioned by Pachinger (p. 187) is surely Saint Expeditus who "expedites" childbirth—a purely verbal creation!

6. This miracle can be found in a note to *PL* 104, col. 251.

7. This miracle has been translated into French by Edmond Albe in *Les Miracles de Notre-Dame de Roc-Amadour au XIIᵉ siècle,* pp. 233–35. I use his translation for my translation into English.

8. For this set of problems see Sigal, *L'Homme et le miracle,* p. 184.

9. Without visible proof many miracles could not officially be recognized.

10. The text is in the *Acta Sanctorum* in the entry for March 20, p. 150. Saint Vulframmus died in 741.

11. The marginal notation for this passage reads, "mirabili apertura corporis liberatur" (he [the baby] is being freed through a miraculous opening of [the mother's] body).

12. *PL* 80, cols. 128–30. The English translation from which I paraphrase and quote is in Garvin, *The "Vitas Sanctorum patrum,"* pp. 161–68, quotations pp. 165, 167.

13. *PL* 80, col. 130.

14. The twelfth-century story, in Latin, and its fourteenth-century transformation, in French, can be found in Gustave Servois, "Notices et extraits du 'Recueil des miracles de Notre-Dame de Rocamadour,'" pp. 38–41.

15. For medieval conceptions of the Virgin as bride or lover, see Warner, *Alone of All Her Sex,* pt. 3.

16. Generally, the texts and images have not been studied together. The woodcuts are mentioned mostly in works on chiroxylographic, xylographic, and early printed books; little attention is given in such works to the texts the woodcuts illustrate. Bing, *Apocalypse Block-Books,* examines the relationship between the block books and their manuscript models. Except for Emmerson, *Antichrist in the Middle Ages* (which says nothing about

Caesarean birth), the major studies on the Antichrist do not mention illustrations. Weindler in *Der Kaiserschnitt*, p. 38, was the only scholar even to speculate on the significance of the Antichrist's birth by Caesarean, but he does so in the vaguest terms ("the Caesarean may signal the birth of a supernatural being"). Just as vague is Zglinicki in *Die Geburt*, p. 131. Schüssler, in "Studien zur Ikonographie des Antichrist," describes several scenes of the Antichrist's birth by Caesarean but is not in the least puzzled by these images. The companion volumes to facsimiles of the German *Entkrist* (cf. Musper, *Der Antichrist*, and Boveland, Burger, and Steffen, *Der Antichrist*) cover just about every angle of the Antichrist's life except his birth by Caesarean, which is so strikingly depicted in these books (figs. 22 and 23). The recent article by McGinn, "Portraying Antichrist," though full of fascinating detail, also contributes nothing to the question of the Antichrist's Caesarean birth.

17. Comprehensive studies on the many theories on the Antichrist's significance for Western culture are Bousset, *Der Antichrist*; Rauh, *Das Bild des Antichrist*; Emmerson.

18. Emmerson, p. 79.

19. Rauh, p. 529.

20. Emmerson, p. 64.

21. Rauh, p. 148.

22. The text and some of its derivations have recently been edited by Verhelst (see Adso Dervensis, *De ortu et tempore Antichristi*). Verhelst demonstrates that the text by Sackur (*Sybillinische Texte . . .*), used by most scholars before 1976, is in fact a composite of different versions.

23. I quote Wright's translation (appended to his translation of the *Ludus de Antichristo*). The scriptural references in brackets are my addition.

24. The Latin text is somewhat ambiguous here: "ex patris et matris copulatione" (lines 31–32). Whether this means "his mother and father" or "his mother and her father" is not quite clear. In any case, the idea of an incestuous relationship between a father and his daughter became prominent later on, especially in vernacular texts (see below the treatment of Berengier's *De l'avènement Antecrist*, Walberg, ed.).

25. This whole passage is also in Bede, *In Apoc.* 17 (*PL* 90, col. 574C).

26. Cf. Haimo of Auxerre (d. 875), *PL* 117, col. 780. Haimo stresses that the Antichrist is the devil's son not "by nature, but by imitation."

27. Cf. Haimo, *PL* 117, col. 780: "Nascetur Antichristus in Babylone de tribu Dan."

28. For details on this text, see Lefèvre, *L'Elucidarium*. Honorius was often called Honorius of Autun, but more recent scholarship identifies "Augustodensis" with a mountainside outside of Regensburg in northern Bavaria.

29. Schorbach, *Studien über das deutsche Volksbuch "Lucidarius,"* p. 7. The spelling of "Endkrist" varies from version to version. I will consistently spell it "Endkrist," except in titles of editions of the "Endkrist" texts.

30. Lerner, *The Heresy of the Free Spirit*, p. 144 n. 45, quotes an amusing dialogue on the ambiguous meaning of the term between two sixteenth-century Germans: "Franz: 'What do you think is the Endchrist? / Karsthans: I really don't know any more than that the priests and the monks preach that he will be a new God and when he comes the world will be destroyed soon after. / Franz: Well, my dear Karsthans, it means something completely different. He is not called Endchrist because he will come at the end of the world, but he is called Ant[i]christ which is a Greek word.'"

31. This is question and answer no. 33; Lefèvre, pp. 453–54.

32. This detail has so far not been noticed. It is a clue to the sources used by the authors of the German *Endkrist* texts: probably not Adso but either Honorius's text or one of its translations.

33. Hildegard of Bingen, *Scivias*, vol. 2, pp. 589–90. Trans. Böckeler, p. 327.

34. The *Compendium theologicae veritatis* was a staple of medieval theology. Written by

Hugo Ripelin of Strasbourg in the thirteenth century, this text was attributed to a large number of different authors such as Thomas Aquinas, Hugh of St. Victor, Albertus Magnus, and Saint Bonaventure. See Steer, *Hugo Ripelin,* for details. There is as yet no critical edition of the text, but one version of it can be found in the Borgnet edition of the complete works of Albertus Magnus (Paris, 1895), vol. 34, p. 241. The Antichrist's birth is described as follows: "Hic ex parentum seminibus concipietur: sed post conceptum descendet spiritus malignus in matris uterum, cujus virtute et operatione deinceps puer nascetur, aletur, adolescet: propter quod filius perditionis vocabitur. Nascetur autem in Babylonia de tribu Dan . . . Post hoc veniet in Jerusalem, et circumcidet se, dicens se esse Christum etc." (He will be conceived from the seeds of the parents. But after the conception the evil spirit descends into the mother's womb. Through his power and acts the boy is born, nourished, and brought up: for this reason he will be called the son of perdition. Thus he will be born in Babylon of the tribe of Dan. . . . After that he will come to Jerusalem where he will be circumcised, claiming that he is Christ).

35. Roy, ed., pp. 219–22.

36. Cf. Schüssler, p. 325. The manuscript is no. 579 of the Municipal Library of Besançon.

37. A facsimile has been edited by Karel Stejskal. See also Antonin Matejcek *Velislova Bible* (Prague: Jan Stenc, 1926). The arrangement of the pages is very similar to that of the German block books: two half-page illustrations with two or three lines of captions.

38. *PL* 117, col. 780B.

39. Ed. Walberg, lines 34–35.

40. *De universo libri XXII,* book 8, chap. 3 (*PL* 111, cols. 228ff.). For the text see Chapter 1, n. 4. The belief in the vipers' strange habits of procreation goes back to the antique tradition of natural history. Galen, for example, quotes some verses from Nicander that state that the viper conceives in the mouth, bites off the male's head, and "the young viper avenges its father's death by gnawing its way out of its mother's vitals" (Thorndike, *History of Magic,* 1:172). For later refutations of this story, see Thorndike, vol. 4, chap. 66: "The Attack on Pliny." The viper's birth was also shown in manuscript illuminations, e.g., in a fourteenth-century manuscript of Bartholomeus Anglicus's *De proprietatibus rerum* (Bibliothèque Ste Geneviève 1029, fol. 262). The shape of the "incision" resembles the incisions seen in images of Caesareans.

41. Ed. Carmody, p. 135.

42. "Pour ce qu'il occist sa mere au naistre." There is no critical edition of this text. The quote comes from manuscript B.N. f. fr. 20316, fol. 312v.

43. Rauh, p. 314.

44. Ibid., p. 350.

45. See Gerhoch von Reichersberg, *Commentarium in Psalmos, PL* 193, col. 821A: "De Babylonia, in quam materiali, seu potius tropica, ut est civitas Roma, dicente Petro: 'Salutat vos Ecclesia in Babylone collecta' (1 Petr. 5:13), quo nomine Romam tropice denotavit."

46. Hind, *Introduction to the History of the Woodcut,* 1:82.

47. *Printing, Selling, and Reading,* p. 4.

48. Bing, p. 152.

49. P. 365.

50. This slit may have been a feature of medieval pregnancy dresses (cf. Alexandre-Bidon and Closson, *L'Enfant,* p. 53). But since the Antichrist's mother is often seen as a parody of the Virgin, one might compare certain representations of the pregnant Virgin, such as Piero della Francesca's *Madonna del Parto* in the cemetery chapel at Monterchi. The Virgin stands upright and points with her right hand to an elongated opening in her blue dress under which a white garment appears. The shape of the opening is more than

suggestive of a Caesarean. A similar dress can be found on a seated Virgin in a fifteenth-century book of hours (B.N. lat. 1174, fol. 69).

51. Lines 454–55.

Appendix   Creative Etymology

1. These questions still preoccupy people today, as can be seen in a *New York Times* article, reflect arguments of a centuries-old debate; it is refreshing to see that some (March 24, 1985), which associated Caesarean birth with Julius Caesar. Several readers raised doubts over this association: Warren Smith from Columbus, Ohio, offered the explanation that the term comes from a law called *lex caesarea;* Morris Silverman from Yeshiva University cited Pliny's *Natural History* and the past participle of *caedere* (to cut), *caesus.* (These letters, printed in the *New York Times* letter section a week after Blakeslee's article, reflect arguments of a centuries-old debate; it is refreshing to see that some questions are as hotly debated today as they were in the Middle Ages.)

2. Zumthor, "Etymologies," p. 147.

3. *European Literature,* p. 495.

4. Ibid., p. 496.

5. *Genealogies and Etymologies,* p. 44.

6. Ibid., p. 48.

7. See below for similar thought processes in medieval historiography.

8. Pundel, *L'Histoire,* p. 17; Trolle, *History of Caesarean Section,* p. 15.

9. Trolle, p. 25.

10. See Pliny, *Natural History,* 7.9, trans. Rackham.

11. Trolle, p. 25.

12. Pundel, p. 18. See Trolle, p. 26, for photographs of this coin.

13. Bloch, p. 57; Isidore of Seville, 9.3.

14. Flutre and Sneyders de Vogel, eds., *Li fet des Romains,* p. 8.

15. *The Twelve Caesars,* trans. Robert Graves, p. 26.

16. For details on the attribution of this translation to Jean du Chesne, see Bossuat, "Traductions françaises."

17. See Flutre, *"Li Faits des Romains,"* and Bossuat.

18. B.N. f. fr. 38, dating from ca. 1482; this manuscript has not yet been edited.

19. In the *Faits* we have an interesting example of creative—and possibly medically informed—translation. None of the Latin texts, including Isidore, the immediate source in this case, indicates that the birth in question was a prolonged one. The translator, however, inserts the word *tant* (such a long time), suggesting an unusually protracted birth, with abdominal delivery as a last resort. In later medical texts tedious labor was indeed listed as one of the indications for a Caesarean. Legends such as that of the Nordic *Volsunga Saga,* which told of a six-year pregnancy ending with a Caesarean, may have been known to the translator and may have suggested a dramatic dimension to the birth quite absent from Isidore. (For the *Saga,* see Diepgen, *Frau und Frauenheilkunde,* p. 55.)

20. Ed. Guy Raynaud and Henri Lemaitre, lines 20454–64.

21. Cf. Benveniste, *Problèmes,* 1:76 and 86.

22. For Mansel see Flutre, *"Li Faits des Romains,"* chap. 8. Mansel's text is as yet unedited.

23. The misattribution of the description of Caesar's birth to Lucan illustrates another phenomenon related to Roman history and the *Faits.* Since the *Faits* was a compilation drawing on a large number of sources without always identifying them, the text as a whole came to stand as a French version of Suetonius, or alternatively a French version of Lucan.

This view persists to this day: two manuscripts listed in the *Catalogue des manuscrits* of the Bibliothèque Nationale in Paris as "Suétone" actually turn out to be manuscripts of the *Faits* (B.N. f. fr. 726 and n. acq. fr. 3650). (They are, however, correctly listed in Flutre, *Les Manuscrits.*) Another manuscript listed as "Commentaire de César" also reveals itself as a *Faits* manuscript (B.N. f. fr. 22540).

24. Soucek, "An Illustrated Manuscript," fig. 3.

25. My thanks go to George Saliba from Columbia University for help with the Arabic.

26. For Alfonso, see *Prosa histórica,* ed. Benito Brancaforte. For *Flos mundi,* see Graf, *Roma,* 1:225.

27. Pp. 62–63.

28. See Gumbrecht, "Literary Translation."

29. Graf, 1:255.

30. For the edition see Schleissner, "Pseudo-Albertus Magnus."

31. Holtzmann, *Geschichte der sächsischen Kaiserzeit,* p. 68, mentions the famous legend that gave Henry the surname *auceps (der Vogler)* but has no details about his birth. Had Henry really been born by Caesarean, this fact would certainly have been mentioned, since it was often construed as an omen for future greatness.

32. This quotation comes from the facsimile edition of the 1513 edition printed in Strasbourg by Martin Flach. Pundel assumes that this "Roman history" refers to Pliny. Since Roesslin does nothing but translate Guy de Chauliac (who most likely refers to the *Faits des Romains*) for this passage, it is useless to speculate what "Roman history" Roesslin had in mind. In any case, Pliny was primarily known not as a Roman historian but as a natural historian.

33. Bernard of Gordon, *Practica sive lilium medicinae,* 7.5; Guy de Chauliac, *Grande chirurgie,* pp. 549–50.

34. See n. 1 for some recent discussions.

BIBLIOGRAPHY

PRIMARY SOURCES

Abulcasis. *La Chirurgie d'Abulcasis*. Trans. L. Leclerc. Paris: J.-B. Baillière, 1861.

Acta sanctorum martii. Vol. 3. Ed. G. Henschenio and D. Paperbrochio. Venice: Baptistam Albrizzi Hieron. Fil. and Sebastian Coleti, 1736.

Adso Dervensis. *De ortu et tempore Antichristi*. Ed. D. Verhelst. Turnholt: Typographi Brepols Editores Pontificii, 1976.

Alba, Ramón. *Del Anticristo*. Madrid: Editora Nacional, 1982.

Albe, Edmond. *Les Miracles de Notre-Dame de Roc-Amadour au XIIe siècle*. Paris: Champion, 1907.

Alfonso el Sabio. *Prosa histórica*. Ed. Benito Brancaforte. Catedra: Letras Hispánicas, 1984.

Argellata, Petrus (Piero) de. *Chirurgia*. Venice: Bonetus Locatellus for Octavianus Scotus, 1497.

Avicenna. *Canon*. Trans. Gerard of Cremona. Venice: Petrus Maufer et Socii, 1486.

Bartholomeus Anglicus. *De proprietatibus rerum*. Lyons: Philippi and Reinhart, 1482.

——. *On the Properties of Things: John Trevisa's Translation of Bartholomeus Anglicus' "De Proprietatibus Rerum": A Critical Text*. 2 vols. Ed. M. C. Seymour. Oxford: Clarendon Press, 1975.

Bauhin, Caspar. "De partu caesareo." In *Gynaeciorum*. 4 vols. Basel: Valdkirch, 1588. Vol. 2, pp. 501–63.

Benedetti, Alessandro. *De re medica*. Basel, 1508.

Bernard of Gordon. *Practica sive lilium medicinae*. Lyons, 1498.

Boguet, Henry. *An Examen of Witches (Discours des sorciers)*. Trans. E. Allen Ashwin. Ed. Montague Summers. London: John Rodker, 1929.

Caelius Aurelianus. *Gynaecia: Fragments of a Latin Version of Soranus' Gynaecia from a Thirteenth-Century Manuscript*. Ed. Miriam and Israel Drabkin. Baltimore: Johns Hopkins University Press, 1951.

Christine de Pizan. *The Book of the City of Ladies*. Trans. Earl Jeffrey Richards. New York: Persea Books, 1982.

Cogliati Arano, Luisa. *Tacuinum sanitatis*. Milan: Electa Editrice. Trans. and ed. Oscar Ratti and Adele Westbrook under the title *The Medieval Health Handbook*. New York: Braziller, 1976.

De Boer, C., ed. *Ovide moralisé*. 5 vols. Verhandelingen der Koninklijke Akademie van Wetenschappen te Amsterdam, vols. 15, 21, 30, 37, 43. Amsterdam: Johannes Mueller, 1915–43.

Deschamps, Eustache. *Le Miroir de mariage*. In *Oeuvres complètes,* vol. 9, ed. Gaston Raynaud. Paris: SATF, 1894.

Eilhart von Oberge. *Tristrant*. Trans. J. W. Thomas. Lincoln: University of Nebraska Press, 1978.

Flutre, L. -F., and K. Sneyders de Vogel, eds. *Li fet des Romains. Compilé ensemble de Salluste, de Suétone et de Lucan*. Paris: Droz, 1936.

Fox, Sally, ed. *The Medieval Woman. An Illuminated Book of Days*. Boston: Little, Brown, 1985.

Garvin, Joseph N. *The "Vitas sanctorum patrum emeretensium": Text and Translation with an Introduction and Commentary*. Washington, D.C.: Catholic University of America Press, 1946.

Gilbertus Anglicus. *Compendium medicinae*. Lyons, 1510.

Goldast, Melchior, ed. *Rerum alamannicarum scriptores*. Frankfurt: Johannes Martinus Porsius, 1661.

Gottfried von Strassburg. *Tristan*. Trans. A. T. Hatto. Harmondsworth: Penguin Books, 1960.

Guillaume de Saint Pathus. *Les Miracles de Saint Louis*. Ed. Percival B. Fay. Paris: Honoré Champion, 1932.

Guy de Chauliac. *La grande chirurgie*. Trans. E. Nicaise. Paris: Félix Alcan, 1890.

Hildegard of Bingen. *Heilkunde*. Trans. Heinrich Schipperges. Salzburg: Otto Müller, 1957.

——. *Scivias*. 2 vols. Ed. Angela Carlevaris and Adelgundis Führkötter. Turnhout: Brepols, 1978.

——. *Scivias, Wisse die Wege*. Trans. Maura Böckeler. Salzburg: Otto Müller, 1954.

Institoris, Heinrich, and Jakob Sprenger. *Malleus maleficarum*. Trans. Montague Summers. London: Pushkin Press, 1948.

——. *Malleus maleficarum*. Trans. Amand Danet under the title *Le marteau des sorcières*. Paris: Plon, 1973.

Jacques (Jacobus) de Voragine. *La Légende dorée*. Trans. J.-B. M. Roze. Paris: Garnier Flammarion, 1967.

Ketsch, Peter. *Frauen im Mittelalter*. 2 vols. Düsseldorf: Schwann-Bagel, 1983.

Lanfranc of Milan, *Science of Surgery*. 2 vols. Ed. Robert von Fleischhacker. Early English Text Society. New York: Scribner's, 1910.

Latini, Brunetto. *Li Livres dou trésor*. Ed. Francis J. Carmody. Berkeley: University of California Press, 1948.

Lefèvre, Yves, ed. *L'Elucidarium et les Lucidaires*. Paris: E. de Boccard, 1954.

The Male Mid-Wife and the Female Doctor: The Gynecology Controversy in Nineteenth-Century America. New York: Arno Press, 1974.

Mason-Hohl, Elizabeth, trans. *The Diseases of Women by Trotula of Salerno: A Translation of the Passionibus mulierum curandorum.* Los Angeles: Ward Ritchie Press, 1940.

Medica antiqua. Libri 4 medicinae. Codex Vindobonensis 93 der österreichischen Nationalbibliothek. Facsimile edition by C. H. Talbot and F. Unterkircher. Graz: Akademische Druck- und Verlagsanstalt, 1972.

Mercurio, Scipione. *La commare o raccoglitrice.* Venice: G. B. Ciotti, 1601.

Moschion. *La gynaecia di Muscione.* Ed. and trans. Rino Radichhi. Pisa: Editi Giardini, 1970.

Muhammad ibn Zakariya, Abu Bkar, al-Razi. *Continens Rasis.* 2 vols. Venice: Octavianus Scotus, 1529.

——. *Kitāb al-Ḥāwī fī al-Ṭibb. An Encyclopedia of Medicine.* 15 vols. Ed. Osmania Oriental Publications Bureau. Hyderabad-Deccan, India, 1955.

Ovid. *Metamorphoses.* With a translation by Frank Justus Miller. 3d ed. Cambridge, Mass.: Harvard University Press, 1977.

Pansier, P. "Un Manuel d'accouchements du XVᵉ siècle." *Janus,* 14 (1909): 217–20.

Paré, Ambroise. *Oeuvres complètes.* Ed. J. F. Malgaigne. Paris: J.-B. Baillière, 1840.

Paulus Aegineta. *The Seven Books.* 3 vols. Trans. Francis Adams. London: Sydenham Society, 1844.

Pliny, *Natural History.* With an English translation by H. Rackham. Cambridge, Mass.: Harvard University Press, 1942.

Pseudo-Methodius. *Opusculum divinarum revelationum.* Ed. Sebastian Brant. Basel, 1498.

Les quinze joies de mariage. Ed. Jean Rychner. Geneva: Droz, 1967.

Rabanus Maurus. *De universo libri XXII. PL* 111.

Rézeau, Pierre. *Les Prières aux saints à la fin du moyen âge.* 2 vols. Geneva: Droz, 1982.

Rhazes. *See* Muhammad ibn Zakariya, Abu Bkar, al-Razi.

Roesslin, Eucharius. *Der Swangern Frawen vnd Hebammen Rosegarten.* Facsimile of the 1513 edition. Zürich: Verlag Bibliophile Drucke, 1976.

Le Roman de Renart le Contrefait. Ed. G. Raynaud and Henri Lemaitre. Paris: Champion, 1914.

Rousset, François. *Traitté nouveau de l'hystérotomotokie, ou enfantement Caesarien.* Paris: Denys du Val, 1581.

Rowland, Beryl, ed. *A Medieval Woman's Guide to Health.* Kent, Ohio: Kent State University Press, 1981.

Roy, Emile, ed. *Le Jour du jugement. Mystère français sur le grand schisme.* Paris, 1902. Reprint. Geneva: Slatkine, 1976.

Sackur, Ernst. *Sybillinische Texte und Forschungen.* Halle: Niemeyer, 1898.

Schleissner, Margaret. "Pseudo-Albertus Magnus. *Secreta mulierum cum commento.* Deutsch. Critical Text and Commentary." Ph.D. diss., Princeton University, 1987.

Seelenwurzgarten. Ulm: Dinckmut, 1483.

Servois, Gustave. "Notices et extraits du 'Recueil des miracles de Notre-Dame de Rocamadour.'" *Bibliothèque de l'Ecole des Chartes,* 4th ser., 18:3 (1857): 8–44.

Soranus of Ephesos. *Soranus' Gynecology.* Trans. Owsei Temkin. Baltimore: Johns Hopkins University Press, 1956.

Suetonius. *The Twelve Caesars*. Trans. Robert Graves. Harmondsworth: Penguin Books, 1980.

Thomas Aquinas. *Summa theologiae*. Ed. and trans. James J. Cunningham. London: Blackfriars, 1975.

Velislai biblia picta. Ed. Karel Stejskal. 2 vols. Prague: Sumptibus Pragopress, 1970.

Vierge et merveille. Les miracles de Notre-Dame narratifs au moyen âge. Textes établis, traduits et présentés par Pierre Kunstmann. Paris: Union Générale d'Editions, 1981.

Virgil. *The Aeneid*. With an English translation by H. R. Fairclough. New and revised ed. 1935. Reprint. Cambridge, Mass.: Harvard University Press 1974.

Walberg, E., ed. *Deux versions inédites de la légende de l'Antéchrist en vers français du XIIIe siècle*. Lund: C. W. K. Gleerup, 1928.

Wickersheimer, Ernest, ed. *Commentaires de la Faculté de Médecine de l'Université de Paris, 1395–1516*. Paris: Imprimerie Nationale, 1915.

Wright, John, trans. *The Play of Antichrist*. Toronto: Pontifical Institute of Mediaeval Studies, 1967.

SECONDARY SOURCES

Alexandre-Bidon, Danièle, and Monique Closson. *L'Enfant à l'ombre des cathédrales*. Lyons: Presses Universitaires de Lyon, 1985.

Alston, Mary Niven. "The Attitude of the Church towards Dissection before 1500." *BHM*, 16 (1944): 221–38.

Amundsen, Darrel W. "Medieval Canon Law on Medical and Surgical Practice by the Clergy." *BHM*, 52 (1978): 22–44.

Anglo, Sydney. "Evident Authority and Authoritative Evidence: The *Malleus Maleficarum*." In Sydney Anglo, ed. *The Damned Art: Essays in the Literature of Witchcraft*. London: Routledge and Kegan Paul, 1977.

Ariès, Philippe. *L'Enfant et la vie familiale sous l'ancien régime*. Paris: Plon, 1960.

Avril, François. *La Librairie de Charles V*. Paris: Bibliothèque Nationale, 1968.

Baroja, Julio Caro. *World of the Witches*. Trans. O.N.V. Glendinning. Chicago: University of Chicago Press, 1964.

Barstow, Anne Llewellyn. "On Studying Witchcraft as Women's History: A Historiography of the the European Witch Persecutions." *Journal of Feminist Studies in Religion*, 4 (1988): 7–19.

Bayon, Henry Peter. "The Masters of Salerno and the Origins of Professional Medical Practice." In Underwood, pp. 203–19. 1953.

Bazala, Vladimir. "Zur Geschichte des Kaiserschnitts." *Grünenthal Waage*, 4 (1965): 61–72.

Becker, Gabriele, et al. *Aus der Zeit der Verzweiflung: Zur Genese und Aktualität des Hexenbildes*. Frankfurt am Main: Suhrkamp Verlag, 1977.

Bell, Enid. *Storming the Citadel: The Rise of the Woman Doctor*. London: Constable, 1953.

Benedek, Thomas G. "The Changing Relationship between Midwives and Physicians during the Renaissance." *BHM*, 51 (1977): 550–64.

Benton, John F. "Trotula, Women's Problems, and the Professionalization of Medicine in the Middle Ages." *BHM*, 59 (1985): 30–53.

Benveniste, Emile. *Problèmes de linguistique générale*. Vol. 1. Paris: Gallimard, 1966.

Bergues, Hélène, et al. *Prévention des naissances dans la famille: Ses origines dans les temps modernes*. Institut national d'études démographiques. Travaux et Documents 35. Paris: Presses Universitaires de France, 1960.

Bing, Gertrud. "The Apocalypse Block-Books and Their Manuscript Models." *Journal of the Warburg and Courtauld Institutes*, 5 (1942): 144–60.

Birkelbach, Dagmar, Christiane Eifert, and Sabine Lueken. "Zur Entwicklung des Hebammenwesens vom 14. bis zum 16. Jahrhundert am Beispiel der Regensburger Hebammenordnungen." In *Frauengeschichte*, pp. 83–98. Dokumentation des 3. Historikerinnentreffens in Bielefeld (April 1981). Munich: Verlag Frauenoffensive, 1981.

Bloch, Howard. *Genealogies and Etymologies: A Literary Anthropology of the French Middle Ages*. Chicago: University of Chicago Press, 1983.

Boss, Jeffrey. "The Antiquity of Caesarean Section with Maternal Survival: The Jewish Tradition." *Medical History*, 5 (1961): 117–31.

Bossuat, Robert. "Traductions françaises des *Commentaires* de César jusqu' à la fin du XVᵉ siècle." *Bibliothèque d'Humanisme et Renaissance*, 3 (1943): 253–411.

Boswell-Stone, W. G. *Shakespeare's Holinshed: The Chronicle and the Historical Plays Compared*. London, 1896. Reprint. New York: Benjamin Blom, 1966.

Bousset, Wilhelm. *Der Antichrist*. Göttingen, 1895. Reprint. New York: Georg Olms, 1983.

Boveland, Karin, Christoph Peter Burger, and Ruth Steffen. *Der Antichrist und die fünfzehn Zeichen vor dem Jüngsten Gericht*. Faksimile Ausgabe und Kommentarband. Hamburg: F. Wittig, 1979.

Brenk, Beat. "Le Texte et l'image dans la *Vie des Saints* au moyen âge: Rôle du concepteur et rôle du peintre." In *Texte et image*, pp. 31–39. 1984.

Brissaud, Y.-B. "L'Infanticide à la fin du moyen âge: Ses motivations psychologiques et sa répression." *Revue Historique de Droit Français et Étranger*, 50 (1972): 229–56.

Brody, S. N. *The Disease of the Soul: Leprosy in Medieval Literature*. Ithaca: Cornell University Press, 1974.

Brundage, James A. *Law, Sex, and Christian Society in Medieval Europe*. Chicago: University of Chicago Press, 1987.

Bullough, Vern. *The Development of Medicine as a Profession*. New York: Hafner, 1966.

——. "The Development of the Medical Guilds at Paris." *Medievalia et Humanistica*, 12 (1958): 33–40.

——. "Female Longevity and Diet in the Middle Ages." *Speculum*, 55 (1980): 315–25.

——. "Medieval Medical and Scientific Views of Women." *Viator*, 4 (1973): 485–501.

——. "Postscript: Heresy, Witchcraft, and Sexuality." In Bullough and Brundage, pp. 206–17. 1982.

Bullough, Vern, and James Brundage, eds. *Sexual Practices and the Medieval Church*. Buffalo: Prometheus Books, 1982.

Carroll, Berenice A., ed. *Liberating Women's History: Theoretical and Critical Essays*. Urbana: University of Illinois Press, 1976.

Carstensen, Gert, Hans Schadewaldt, and Paul Vogt. *Die Chirurgie in der Kunst.* Düsseldorf: Econ, 1983.

Cash, Arthur H. "The Birth of Tristram Shandy: Sterne and Dr. Burton." In R. R. Brissenden, ed. *Studies in the Eighteenth Century: Papers Presented at the David Nicholl Smith Seminar 1966,* pp. 133–54. Canberra: Australian National University Press, 1968.

Clarke, Edwin, ed. *Modern Methods in the History of Medicine.* London: Athlone Press, 1971.

Coleman, Emily. "Infanticide in the Early Middle Ages." In Stuard, pp. 47–70. 1976.

Cornell, Henrik. *The Iconography of the Nativity of Christ.* Uppsala: A.-B. Lundequistska Bokhandeln, 1924.

Cosman, Madeleine Pelner. "Medieval Medical Malpractice: The Dicta and the Dockets." In Saul Jarcho, ed. *Essays and Notes on the History of Medicine,* pp. 71–96. New York: New York Academy of Medicine, 1976.

Coulton, George. *Life in the Middle Ages.* 4 vols. Cambridge: Cambridge University Press, 1930.

Curschmann, Michael. "Hören—Sehen—Lesen. Buch und Schriftlichkeit im Selbstverständnis der volkssprachlichen literarischen Kultur Deutschlands um 1200." *Beiträge zur Geschichte der deutschen Sprache und Literatur,* 106 (1984): 218–57.

Curtius, Ernst Robert. *European Literature and the Latin Middle Ages.* Trans. Willard R. Trask. Bollingen series. Princeton: Princeton University Press, 1973.

Davis, Natalie Zemon. "Gender and Genre: Women as Historical Writers, 1400–1820." In Labalme, pp. 153–82. 1980.

Delaissé, L. M. J. *La Miniature flamande: Le mécénat de Philippe le Bon.* Brussels: Palais des Beaux Arts, 1959.

Demaitre, Luke. *Doctor Bernard de Gordon: Professor and Practitioner.* Toronto: Pontifical Institute of Mediaeval Studies, 1980.

——. "The Idea of Childhood and Child Care in Medical Writings of the Middle Ages." *Journal of Psychohistory,* 4 (1977): 461–90.

——. "Scholasticism in the Compendia of Practical Medicine, 1250–1450." *Manuscripta,* 20 (1976): 81–95.

——. "Theory and Practice in Medical Education at the University of Montpellier in the Thirteenth and Fourteenth Centuries." *JHM,* 30 (1975): 103–23.

Demats, Paule. *Fabula. Trois études de mythographie antique et médiévale.* Geneva: Droz, 1973.

DeMause, Lloyd, ed. *The History of Childhood.* New York: Psychohistory Press, 1974.

Diepgen, Paul. *Frau und Frauenheilkunde in der Kultur des Mittelalters.* Stuttgart: Georg Thieme, 1963.

Donegan, Jane B. *Women and Men Midwives: Medicine, Morality, and Misogyny in Early America.* Westport, Conn.: Greenwood Press, 1978.

Donnison, Jean. *Midwives and Medical Men: A History of Interprofessional Rivalries and Women's Rights.* London: Heinemann, 1978.

Eccles, Audrey. *Obstetrics and Gynaecology in Tudor and Stuart England.* Kent, Ohio: Kent State University Press, 1982.

Ehrenreich, Barbara, and Deirdre English. *Witches, Midwives, and Nurses: A History of Women Healers.* Westbury, N.Y.: Feminist Press, 1973.

Emmerson, Richard Kenneth. *Antichrist in the Middle Ages: A Study of Medieval Apocalypticism, Art, and Literature.* Seattle: University of Washington Press, 1981.

Ennen, Edith. *Frauen im Mittelalter.* Munich: C. H. Beck, 1984.

Farquhar, James Douglas, and Sandra Hindman. *Pen to Press: Illustrated Manuscripts and Printed Books in the First Century of Printing.* College Park: Art Department, University of Maryland, 1977.

Fasbender, Heinrich. *Geschichte der Geburtshilfe.* Jena: Gustav Fischer, 1906.

Feis, Oswald. "Bericht aus dem Jahre 1411 über eine Hebamme, die angeblich sieben Kaiserschnitte mit gutem Erfolg für Mutter und Kind ausgeführt hat." *Sudhoffs Archiv für Geschichte der Medizin,* 26 (1933): 340–43.

Ferrante, Joan. "The Education of Women in the Middle Ages in Theory, Fact, and Fantasy." In Labalme, pp. 1–42. 1980.

Flandrin, L. "Contraception, mariage, et relations amoureuses dans l'occident chrétien." *Annales. Economies, Sociétés, Civilisations,* 24 (1969): 1370–90.

Flutre, L. -F. "Encore un manuscrit des 'Faits des Romains.'" *Neophilologus,* 19 (1933–34): 95; 21 (1935–36): 19–21.

——. *"Li Faits des Romains" dans les littératures française et italienne du XIIIe au XVIe siècle.* Paris: Hachette, 1932.

——. *Les Manuscrits des "Faits des Romains."* Paris: Hachette, 1932.

——. "La Naissance de César." *Aesculape,* 24 (1934): 244–50.

Forbes, Thomas. *The Midwife and the Witch.* New Haven: Yale University Press, 1966.

——. "Midwifery and Witchcraft." *JHM,* 17 (1962): 264–83.

Forsyth, Ilene H. "Children in Early Medieval Art: Ninth through Twelfth Centuries." *Journal of Psychohistory,* 4:1 (1976): 31–70.

Foucault, Michel. *La Naissance de la clinique.* Paris: Presses Universitaires de France, 1963.

Freeman, Jo, ed. *Women: A Feminist Perspective.* Palo Alto: Mayfield Publishing, 1975.

Friedländer, Max. *Der Holzschnitt.* 4th ed. Berlin: De Gruyter, 1970.

Gall, Piero. *L'iconografia del taglio cesareo.* Monografie Ostetrico-Ginecologiche. Milan, 1936.

Gélis, Jacques. "La Formation des accoucheurs et des sages-femmes aux XVIIe et XVIIIe siècles." *Annales de démographie historique,* 1977: 153–80.

Glesinger, L. "La Naissance de Vopiscus Fortunatus Plempius." *Scalpel,* 108 (1955): 673–78.

Goff, Frederick. *Incunabula in American Libraries.* New York: Bibliographical Society of America, 1964.

Gold, Penny Schine. *The Lady and the Virgin: Image, Attitude, and Experience in Twelfth-Century France.* Chicago: The University of Chicago Press, 1985.

Gombrich, E. H. *Art and Illusion: A Study in the Psychology of Pictorial Representation.* The A. W. Mellon Lectures in the Fine Arts, 1956. Bollingen Series 35:5. Princeton: Princeton University Press, 1969.

Graf, Arturo. *Roma nella memoria e nelle imaginazioni del medio evo.* 2 vols. Torino: Ermanno Loescher, 1882.

Grape-Albers, Heide. *Spätantike Bilder aus der Welt des Arztes. Medizinische Bilder-*

handschriften der Spätantike und ihre mittelalterliche Überlieferung. Wiesbaden: G. Pressler, 1977.

Green, Monica Helen. "Toward a History of Women's Medical Practice and Medical Care in Medieval Europe." *Signs,* 14 (1989):434–73.

——. "The Transmission of Ancient Theories of Female Physiology and Disease through the Early Middle Ages." Ph.D. diss., Princeton University, 1985.

Gubalke, Wolfgang. *Die Hebamme im Wandel der Zeiten.* Frankfurt: Staude, 1964.

Guénée, Bernard. "La Culture historique des nobles: Le succès des *Faits des Romains* (XIIIᵉ–XVᵉ siècle)." In Philippe Contamine, ed., *La Noblesse au moyen âge,* pp. 261–88. Paris: Presses Universitaires de France, 1976.

Gumbrecht, H. U. "Literary Translation and Its Social Conditioning in the Middle Ages: Four Spanish Romance Texts of the Thirteenth Century." *Yale French Studies,* 51 (1974): 205–22.

Guyonnet, Georges. "Quelques grands conflits foeto-maternels historiques et légendaires." *Aesculape,* 39 (1956): 46–64.

Hammond, E. A. "Incomes of Medieval English Doctors." *JHM,* 15 (1960): 154–69.

Hanawalt, Barbara A., ed. *Women and Work in Preindustrial Europe.* Bloomington: Indiana University Press, 1986.

Hansen, Joseph. *Quellen und Untersuchungen zur Geschichte des Hexenwahns und der Hexenverfolgungen im Mittelalter.* Bonn, 1901. Reprint. Hildesheim: Georg Olms, 1963.

——. *Zauberwahn, Inquisition, und Hexenprozess im Mittelalter und die Entstehung der grossen Hexenverfolgung.* Munich: R. Oldenbourg, 1900.

Harksen, Sibylle. *Die Frau im Mittelalter.* Leipzig: Edition Leipzig, 1974.

Hartge, R. "Nur die Götter kamen wunderbar zur Welt." *Grünenthal Waage,* 16 (1977): 259–64.

Hefele, Carl Joseph von. *Conciliengeschichte.* Freiburg: Herder'sche Verlagshandlung, 1890.

Hefele, Carl Joseph von, and H. Leclercq. *Histoire des Conciles.* 11 vols. Paris: Letouzey et Ané, 1907–52.

Heinsohn, Gunnar, and Otto Steiger. *Die Vernichtung der weisen Frauen. Hexenverfolgung. Menschenproduktion. Kinderwelten. Bevölkerungswissenschaft. Beiträge zur Theorie und Geschichte von Bevölkerung und Kindheit.* Herbstein: März, 1985.

Herlihy, David. "Life Expectancies for Women in Medieval Society." In Morewedge, pp. 1–22. 1975.

Herrlinger Robert. *Geschichte der medizinischen Abbildung.* 2 vols. Munich: Heinz Moos, 1967.

Hind, Arthur M. *An Introduction to the History of the Woodcut.* 2 vols. 1935. Reprint. New York: Dover Publications, 1963.

Hirsch, Rudolf. *Printing, Selling, and Reading: 1450–1550.* Wiesbaden: Otto Harrassowitz, 1974.

Holländer, Eugen. *Die Medizin in der klassischen Malerei.* Stuttgart: Ferdinand Enke, 1923.

Holtzmann, Robert. *Geschichte der sächsischen Kaiserzeit, 900–1024.* Munich: Georg D. W. Callwey, 1946.

Horsley, Ritta Jo, and Richard A. Horsley. "On the Trail of the 'Witches': Wise

Women, Midwives, and the European Witch Hunts." In Marianne Burkhard and Edith Waldstein, eds., *Women in German Yearbook 3,* pp. 1–28. Lanham, Md.: University Press of America, 1986.

Huard, P., and M. D. Grmek. *Mille ans de chirurgie en occident: V^e–XVe siècles.* Paris: Dacosta, 1966.

Hughes, Muriel. *Women Healers in Medieval Life and Literature.* 1943. Reprint. New York: Books for Libraries, 1968.

Hunt, David. *Parents and Children in History.* New York: Basic Books, 1970.

Hurd-Mead, Kate Campbell. *A History of Women in Medicine.* Haddam, Conn.: Haddam Press, 1938.

Imbault-Huart, M. -J. *La Médecine médiévale à travers les manuscrits de la Bibliothèque Nationale.* Paris: Bibliothèque Nationale, 1982.

Jacobsen, Grethe. "Pregnancy and Childbirth in the Medieval North: A Typology of Sources and a Preliminary Study." *Scandinavian Journal of History,* 9 (1984): 91–111.

Jacquart, Danielle. *Le Milieu médical en France du XIIe au XVe siècle.* Hautes Etudes Médiévales et Modernes 46. Geneva: Droz, 1981.

——. *Supplément au dictionnaire de Wickersheimer.* Vol. 3 of the reprint ed. of Wickersheimer's *Dictionnaire.* Geneva: Droz, 1979.

Jacquart, Danielle, and Claude Thomasset. *Sexualité et savoir médical au moyen âge.* Paris: Presses Universitaires de France, 1985.

Jones, Peter Murray. *Medieval Medical Miniatures.* Austin: University of Texas Press, 1985.

Kealy, Edward J. *Medieval Medicus.* Baltimore: Johns Hopkins University Press, 1981.

Kelchner, Ernst. *Der Enndkrist.* Frankfurt: Verlag der Frankfurter Lichtdruckanstalt, Wiesbaden, 1891.

Keupper Valle, Rosemary. "The Cesarean Operation in Alta California During the Franciscan Mission Period." *BHM,* 48 (1974): 265–75.

Kibre, Pearl. "The Faculty of Medicine at Paris, Charlatanism, and Unlicensed Medical Practices in the Later Middle Ages." *BHM,* 27 (1953): 1–20.

Kieckhefer, Richard. *European Witch Trials.* Berkeley: University of California Press, 1976.

Kirchner, Josef. *Die Darstellung der ersten Menschenpaares in der Kunst.* Stuttgart: Ferdinand Enke, 1903.

Kirshner, Julius, and Suzanne F. Wemple, eds. *Women of the Medieval World.* Essays in Honor of John H. Mundy. New York: Basil Blackwell, 1985.

Klaits, Joseph. *Servants of Satan: The Age of the Witch Hunts.* Bloomington: Indiana University Press, 1985.

Kristeller, Paul. *Kupferstich und Holzschnitt in vier Jahrhunderten.* 4th ed. Berlin: B. Cassirer, 1922.

Kurz, Otto. "The Medical Illustrations of the Wellcome MS." In Saxl 1942, pp. 137–42.

Labalme, Patricia H., ed. *Beyond Their Sex: Learned Women of the European Past.* New York: New York University Press, 1980.

Labarge, Margaret Wade. *A Small Sound of the Trumpet: Women in Medieval Life.* London: Hamish Hamilton, 1986.

Laget, Mireille. "La Césarienne ou la tentation de l'impossible, XVIIᵉ et XVIIIᵉ siècle." *Annales de Bretagne et des Pays de l'Ouest,* 86 (1979): 177–89.

——. "Childbirth in Seventeenth- and Eighteenth-Century France: Obstetrical Practices and Collective Attitudes." In Robert Forster and Orest Ranum, eds., *Medicine and Society in France,* pp. 137–76. Baltimore: Johns Hopkins University Press, 1980.

——. *Naissances. L'accouchement avant l'âge de la clinique.* Paris: Seuil, 1982.

Lehmann, Volker. *Die Geburt in der Kunst. Geburtshilfliche Motive in der darstellenden Kunst in Europa von der Antike bis zur Gegenwart.* Braunschweig: Braunschweiger Verlagsanstalt, 1978.

Leifer, Myra. "Pregnancy." In Stimpson and Person, pp. 212–23. 1980.

Lemay, Helen Rodnite. "Anthonius Guainerius and Medieval Gynecology." In Kirshner and Wemple, pp. 317–36. 1985.

Lerner, Robert, E. *The Heresy of the Free Spirit in the Later Middle Ages.* Berkeley: University of California Press, 1972.

Levens, H. E., and H. Sinz. *Die künstliche Geburt. Eine illustrierte Geschichte des Kaiserschnitts.* Basel: Sandoz, 1967.

Lindberg, David C., ed. *Science in the Middle Ages.* Chicago: University of Chicago Press, 1978.

Lipinska, Melanie. *Histoire des femmes médecins.* Paris: G. Jacques, 1900.

Macfarlane, Alan. *Witchcraft in Tudor and Stuart England.* New York: Harper and Row, 1970.

McGinn, Bernard, "Portraying Antichrist in the Middle Ages." In Werner Verbeke, Daniel Verhelst, and Andries Welkenhuysen, eds., *The Use and the Abuse of Eschatology,* pp. 1–48. Mediaevalia Lovaniensia, Series 1, Studia 15. Leuven: Leuven University Press, 1988.

MacKinney, Loren C. "Childbirth in the Middle Ages as Seen in Manuscript Illustrations." *Ciba Symposium,* 8 (1960): 230–36.

——. *Early Medieval Medicine with Special Reference to France and Chartres.* Baltimore: Johns Hopkins University Press, 1937.

——. "Medical Education in the Middle Ages." *Cahiers d'Histoire Mondiale,* 2.4 (1955): 835–61.

——. *Medical Illustrations in Medieval Manuscripts.* London: Wellcome Historical Library, 1965.

——. "A Thirteenth-Century Medical Case History in Miniatures." *Speculum,* 35 (1960): 251–59.

McLaughlin, Mary Martin. "Survivors and Surrogates: Children and Parents from the Ninth to the Thirteenth Centuries." In DeMause, pp. 101–81. 1974.

McNamara, Jo Ann. "Chaste Marriage and Clerical Celibacy." In Bullough and Brundage, pp. 22–33. 1982.

McVaugh, Michael. "History of Medicine." In *The Dictionary of the Middle Ages,* 8:247–54. New York: Scribner's, 1987.

Meier, Christel, and U. Ruberg. *Text und Bild.* Wiesbaden: L. Reichert, 1980.

Metz, René. *La Femme et l'enfant dans le droit canonique médiéval.* London: Variorum Reprints, 1985.

Meyer, Paul. "Les premières compilations françaises d'histoire ancienne." *Romania,* 14 (1885): 1–81.

Midelfort, H. C. Erik. *Witch Hunting in Southwestern Germany, 1562–1684: The Social and Intellectual Foundations*. Stanford: Stanford University Press, 1972.

Miles, Margaret R. *Image as Insight*. Boston: Beacon Press, 1985.

Monter, E. William. *Witchcraft in France and Switzerland: The Borderlands during the Reformation*. Ithaca: Cornell University Press, 1976.

Moore, Robert Ian. *The Formation of a Persecuting Society in Western Europe, 950–1250*. Oxford: Blackwell, 1987.

Morewedge, Rosemarie Thee, ed. *The Role of Women in the Middle Ages*. Albany: State University of New York Press, 1975.

Morton, Leslie Thomas. *A Medical Bibliography (Garrison-Morton): An Annotated Check-List of Texts Illustrating the History of Medicine*. 4th ed. Aldershot: Gower, 1983.

Müllerheim, R. *Die Wochenstube in der Kunst*. Stuttgart: Ferdinand Enke, 1904.

Musper, H. Th., ed. *Der Antichrist und die fünfzehn Zeichen*. Munich: Prestel, 1970.

Nelson, Mary. "Why Witches Were Women." In Freeman, pp. 335–50. 1975.

Newell, Franklin S. *Cesarean Section*. New York: D. Appleton, 1921.

Noonan, John T. *Contraception: A History of Its Treatment by Catholic Theologians and Canonists*. Enlarged ed. Cambridge, Mass.: Harvard University Press, 1986.

O'Malley, C. D. *The History of Medical Education*. UCLA Forum in Medical Sciences 12. Berkeley: University of California Press, 1970.

Oppenheim, Leo A. "A Caesarian Section in the Second Millenium B.C." *JHM*, 15 (1960): 292–94.

Otis, Leah L. "Municipal Wet Nurses in Fifteenth-Century Montpellier." In Hanawalt, pp. 83–93. 1986.

Ouerd, Michèle. "Dans la forge à cauchemars mythologiques. Sorcières, praticiennes et hystériques." *Cahiers de Fontenay*, 11–12 (1985–86): 139–214.

Pachinger, Anton Max. *Die Mutterschaft in der Malerei und Graphik*. Munich: G. Müller, 1906.

Paravy, Pierrette. "L'Angoisse collective au seuil de la mort: résurrections et baptêmes d'enfants mort-nés en Dauphiné au XVᵉ siècle." In *La Mort au moyen âge*, pp. 87–102. Colloque de la société des historiens médiévistes de l'enseignement supérieur public. Publications de la société savante de l'Alsace et des régions de l'est. Collection "Recherches et Documents," 25. Strasbourg: Librairie Istra, 1975.

Park, Katherine. *Doctors and Medicine in Early Renaissance Florence*. Princeton: Princeton University Press, 1985.

Payer, Pierre. *Sex and the Penitentials: The Development of a Sexual Code, 550–1150*. Toronto: University of Toronto Press, 1984.

Pecker, André, and Henri Roulland. *L'Accouchement au cours des siècles*. Paris: Dacosta, 1958.

Peters, Edward. *The Magician, the Witch, and the Law*. Philadelphia: University of Pennsylvania Press, 1978.

Petrelli, Richard L. "The Regulation of French Midwifery during the *Ancien Régime*." *JHM*, 26 (1971): 276–92.

Pfister, Kurt, E. *Das Puch von dem Entkrist*. Leipzig: Insel, 1925.

Pickering, F. P. *Literatur und darstellende Kunst im Mittelalter*. Berlin: Erich Schmidt, 1966.

Porcher, Jean. *Manuscrits à peintures du XIIIe au XVIe siècle*. Paris: Bibliothèque Nationale, 1955.

Pouchelle, Marie-Christine. *Corps et chirurgie à l'apogée du moyen âge*. Paris: Flammarion, 1983.

——. "La Prise en charge de la mort: Médecine, médecins et chirurgiens devant les problèmes liés à la mort à la fin du Moyen Age (XIIIe–XVe siècles)." *Archives Européennes de Sociologie*, 17 (1976): 249–78.

Pundel, J. *L'Histoire de l'opération césarienne. Etude historique de la césarienne dans la médecine, l'art et la littérature, les religions et la législation*. Brussels: Presses Académiques Européennes, 1969.

Rauh, Horst Dieter. *Das Bild des Antichrist im Mittelalter: Von Tyconius zum deutschen Symbolismus*. Münster: Aschendorff, 1979.

Richter, Erwin. "Die Opferung eiserner Bärmutterkrötenvotive im schwäbischen Sonderkult des heiligen Rochus als himmlischer Gynäkologe." *Württembergisches Jahrbuch für Volkskunde*, 1959–60:72–92.

Riddle, John M. "Theory and Practice in Medieval Medicine." *Viator*, 5 (1977): 157–84.

Riesmann, David. *The Story of Medicine in the Middle Ages*. New York: Hoebner, 1935.

Roberts, R. S. "The Use of Literary and Documentary Evidence in the History of Medicine." In Clarke, pp. 36–56. 1971.

Rosenberg, Charles E. "The Medical Profession, Medical Practice, and the History of Medicine." In Clarke, pp. 22–35. 1971.

Rosenthal, Carl Oskar. "Zur geburtshilflich-gynäkologischen Betätigung des Mannes bis zum Ausgange des 16. Jahrhunderts." *Janus*, 27 (1923): 117–48 and 192–212.

Rousselle, A. "La Sage-femme et le thaumaturge dans la Gaule tardive." *Revue Archéologique Centre France*, 22 (1983): 261–71.

Rowland, Beryl. *Birds with Human Souls: A Guide to Bird Symbolism*. Knoxville: University of Tennessee Press, 1978.

Russell, Jeffrey Burton. *Witchcraft in the Middle Ages*. Ithaca: Cornell University Press, 1972.

Salomon, Richard. *Opicinus de Canistris. Weltbild und Bekenntnisse eines avignonesischen Klerikers des 14. Jahrhunderts*. 2 vols. London: Warburg Institute, 1936.

Salvat, Michel. "L'Accouchement dans la littérature scientifique médiévale." In *L'Enfant au moyen âge*, pp. 89–106. Senefiance 9. Aix-en-Provence: CUER, 1980.

Sanchez Arcas, R. "Contribución al estudio histórico e iconográfico de la operación cesarea." *Medicina e Historia*, 25 (1966).

——. "Creencias, supersticiónes y mitos que fueron considerados inhibidores y facilitadores de la parturición." *Medicina e Historia*, 72 (1970).

——. "Datos históricos sobre la operación cesarea: Rousset y su obra (siglo XVI)." *Medicina e Historia*, 38 (1967).

Saxl, Fritz. "A Spiritual Encyclopedia of the Later Middle Ages." *Journal of the Courtauld and Warburg Institutes*, 5 (1942): 82–137.

Schorbach, Karl. *Studien über das deutsche Volksbuch "Lucidarius" und seine Bearbeitungen in fremden Sprachen*. Strasbourg: Karl Trübner, 1894.

Schreiber, Wilhelm L. *Handbuch der Holz- und Metallschnitte des 15. Jahrhunderts.* 11 vols. Leipzig: Hiersemann, 1926–30.

Schroeder, Horst. *Der Topos der Nine Worthies in Literatur und bildender Kunst.* Göttingen: Vandenhoeck and Ruprecht, 1971.

Schüssler, Gosbert. "Studien zur Ikonographie des Antichrist." Diss., Heidelberg, 1975.

Shahar, Shulamith. *The Fourth Estate: A History of Women in the Middle Ages.* Trans. Chaya Galai. London: Methuen, 1983.

——. *Die Frau im Mittelalter.* Trans. Ruth Achlama. Koenigstein: Athenäum, 1981.

Sigal, Pierre-André. *L'Homme et le miracle dans la France médiévale (XIᵉ–XIIᵉ siècle).* Paris: Cerf, 1985.

Singer, Charles. *The Evolution of Anatomy.* London: Kegan Paul, Trench, Trubner, 1925.

——. "Thirteenth-Century Miniatures Illustrating Medical Practice." *Proceedings of the Royal Society of Medicine,* 9 (1916): 29–42.

Siraisi, Nancy G. *Taddeo Alderotti and His Pupils: Two Generations of Italian Medical Learning.* Princeton: Princeton University Press, 1981.

Smith, Hilda. "Gynecology and Ideology in Seventeenth-Century England." In Carroll, pp. 97–114. 1976.

Soucek, P. "An Illustrated Manuscript of al-Bīrūnī's *Chronology of Ancient Nations.*" In Peter J. Chelkowski, ed. *The Scholar and the Saint,* pp. 103–68. New York: New York University Press, 1975.

Speert, Harold. *Iconographia Gyniatrica.* Philadelphia: F. A. Davis, 1973.

Steer, Georg. *Hugo Ripelin von Strassburg: Zur Rezeptions- und Wirkungsgeschichte des "Compendium theologicae veritatis" im deutschen Spätmittelalter.* Tübingen: Max Niemeyer, 1981.

Stimpson, Catharine, and Ethel Spector Person, eds. *Women: Sex and Sexuality.* Chicago: University of Chicago Press, 1980.

Stock, Brian. *The Implications of Literacy: Written Language and Models of Interpretation in the Eleventh and Twelfth Centuries.* Princeton: Princeton University Press, 1983.

Stuard, Susan Mosher, ed. *Women in Medieval Society.* Philadelphia: University of Pennsylvania Press, 1976.

Sudhoff, Karl. *Beiträge zur Geschichte der Chirurgie im Mittelalter. Graphische und textliche Untersuchungen in mittelalterlichen Handschriften.* Studien zur Geschichte der Medizin 10–12. Leipzig, 1914–18.

——. "Die Salernitaner Handschrift in Breslau." *Archiv für Geschichte der Medizin,* 12 (1920): 101–48.

Talbot, Charles H. "Medical Education in the Middle Ages." In O'Malley, pp. 73–87. 1970.

——. "Medicine." In Lindberg, pp. 391–428. 1978.

——. *Medicine in Medieval England.* London: Oldbourne, 1967.

Temkin, Owsei. "The Historiography of Ideas in Medicine." In Clarke, pp. 1–21. 1971.

Texte et image. Actes du Colloque International de Chantilly, 13–15 October 1982. Paris: Les Belles Lettres, 1984.

Thomas, Keith. *Religion and the Decline of Magic.* New York: Scribner's, 1971.

Thomasset, Claude. "Quelques principes de l'embryologie médiévale (de Salerne à la fin du XIIIᵉ siècle)." In *L'Enfant au moyen âge*, pp. 109–21. Senefiance 9. Aix-en-Provence: CUER, 1980.

Thorndike, Lynn. *A History of Magic and Experimental Science*. 8 vols. New York: Columbia University Press, 1923–58.

Thornton, John L., and Carole Reeves. *Medical Book Illustration*. New York: Oleander Press, 1983.

Torpin, Richard, and Iraj Vafaie. "The Birth of Rustam: An Early Account of Caesarean Section in Iran." *American Journal of Obstetrics and Gynecology*, 81.1 (1961): 185–89.

Towler, Jean, and Joan Bramall. *Midwives in History and Society*. London: Croom Helm, 1986.

Trexler, Richard C. "Infanticide in Florence: New Sources and First Results." *History of Childhood Quarterly*, 1 (1973–74): 98–116.

Trolle, Dyre. *The History of Caesarean Section*. Copenhagen: C. A. Reitzel, 1982.

Ullmann, Manfred. *Die Medizin im Islam*. Leiden: Brill, 1970.

Underwood, E. A., ed. *Science, Medicine, and History. Essays on the Evolution of Scientific Thought and Medical Practice Written in Honour of Charles Singer*. New York: Oxford University Press, 1953.

Vercauteren, F. "Les Médecins dans les principautés de la Belgique et du Nord de la France." *Le Moyen Age*, 57 (1951): 61–92.

Warner, Marina. *Alone of All Her Sex: The Myth and the Cult of the Virgin Mary*. 1976. New York: Vintage Books, 1983.

Weindler, Fritz. *Geschichte der gynäkologisch-anatomischen Abbildung*. Dresden: Zahn and Jaensch, 1908.

——. "Der Kaiserschnitt nach den ältesten Überlieferungen unter Zugrundelegung von 18 Geburtsdarstellungen." *Janus*, 20 (1915): 1–20.

Weinstein, Donald, and Rudolph M. Bell, *Saints and Society: The Two Worlds of Western Christendom, 1000–1700*. Chicago: University of Chicago Press, 1982.

Wetherbee, Winthrop. *Platonism and Poetry: The Literary Influence of the School of Chartres*. Princeton: Princeton University Press, 1972.

Wickersheimer, Ernest. *Dictionnaire biographique des médecins en France au moyen âge*. 3 vols. Reprint. Geneva: Droz 1979.

Wieck, R. S. *Late Medieval and Renaissance Illuminated Manuscripts (1350–1525) in the Houghton Library*. Cambridge, Mass.: Department of Printing and Graphic Arts, Harvard College Library, 1983.

Wiesner, Merry. "Early Modern Midwifery: A Case Study." In Hanawalt, pp. 94–113. 1986.

Wilson, Adrian. "Participant or Patient? Seventeenth Century Childbirth from the Mother's Point of View." In Roy Porter, ed. *Patients and Practitioners: Lay Perceptions of Medicine in Preindustrial Society*, pp. 129–44. Cambridge: Cambridge University Press, 1985.

Woledge, Brian. "Encore des manuscrits des *Faits des Romains*." *Neophilologus*, 24 (1938–39): 39–42.

——. "Un manuscrit des *Faits des Romains*." *Romania*, 59 (1933): 564–66.

Wyman, A. L. "The Surgeoness: The Female Practitioner of Surgery, 1400–1800." *Medical History,* 28 (1984): 22–41.

Wyss, R. L. *Die Caesarteppiche und ihr ikonographisches Verhältnis zur Illustration der "Faits des Romains" im 14. und 15. Jahrhundert.* Berner Schriften zur Kunst 9. Bern: Bernisches Historisches Museum, 1957.

Young, John H. *Caesarean Section: The History and Development of the Operation from Earliest Times.* London: H. K. Lewis, 1944.

Zglinicki, Friedrich von. *Geburt: Eine Kulturgeschichte in Bildern.* Braunschweig: Westermann, 1983.

Zilboorg, Gregory. *The Medical Man and the Witch during the Renaissance.* Baltimore: Johns Hopkins University Press, 1935.

Zumthor, Paul. "Etymologies." In *Langue, texte, énigme,* pp. 144–60. Paris: Editions du Seuil, 1975.

INDEX

Library of Congress Cataloging-in-Publication Data

Blumenfeld-Kosinki, Renate, 1952–
    Not of woman born: representations of caesarean birth in medieval and Renaissance culture / Renate Blumenfeld-Kosinski.
        p.   cm.
    Includes bibliographical references.
    ISBN 0-8014-2292-2
        1. Cesarean section—Europe—History.   2. Cesarean section in art.
    3. Medical illustration—History.   4. Civilization, Medieval.
    5. Renaissance.   I. Title.
    RG761.B48 1990
    618.8'6'0902—dc20

                                                89-17421